MEDICAL WISDOM

THE KNOWLEDGE YOU NEED TO NAVIGATE LIFE'S MEDICAL SITUATIONS

By

Mark Borden MD

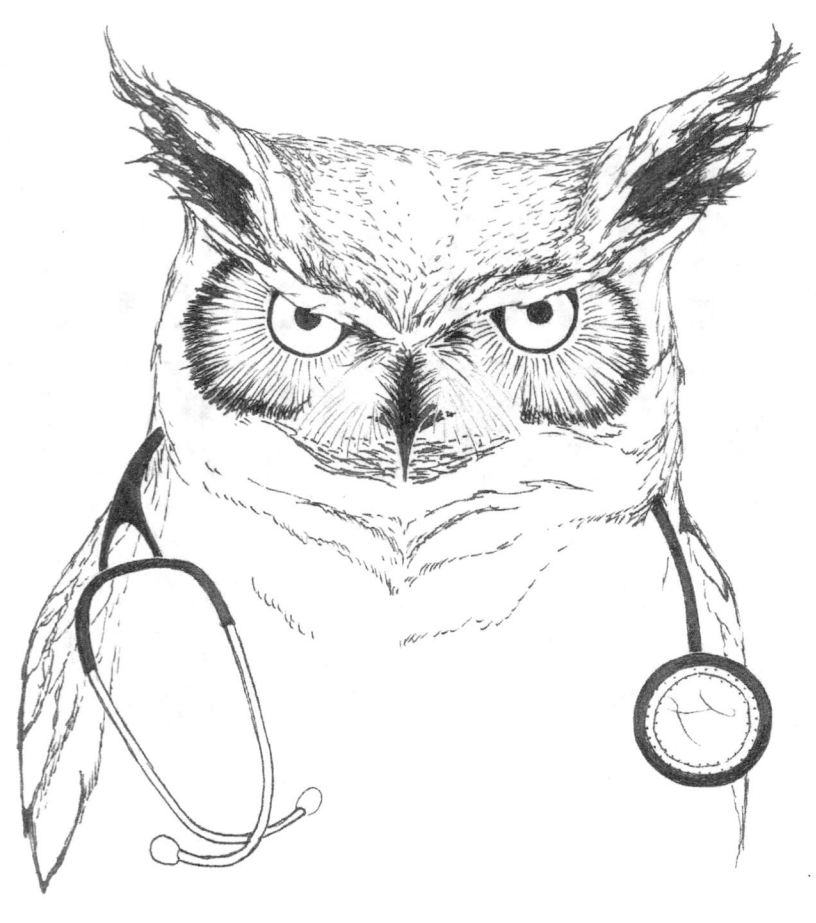

The owl, a symbol of wisdom.

Illustrations by Mary Ellen Oconnor of Whidbey Island Washington

Copyright © 2012, 2017 Mark Borden MD
All rights reserved.
ISBN: 1477461930
ISBN 13: 9781477461938

Disclaimer

Contents

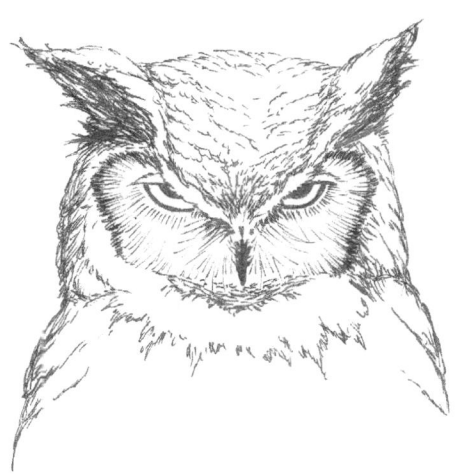

Medical Wisdom

Always remember the simplicity of wisdom in our world of complex knowledge.

—Ron Young

Introduction

Always remember the simplicity of wisdom in our world of complex knowledge.

—Ron Young

What is wisdom? The American Heritage Dictionary defines wisdom as: "1. Understanding of what is true, right, or lasting. 2. Common sense; sagacity; good judgment. 'It is a characteristic of wisdom not to do desperate things' (Thoreau). 3. Learning; erudition…"

The first definition contains several important points: Wisdom should have a permanent quality. New medicines come and go, but what we are trying to accomplish with those medicines remains. Understanding the true goal of treatment allows a person, whether doctor or patient, to know if a medicine is working. In the "Hypertension" chapter we will discuss the treatment of high blood pressure. Any fool can prescribe or take pills to lower a blood pressure number. A wise doctor (and patient) realizes that the goal is not to lower a number, but to reduce the risk of the medical problems that result from high blood pressure, and more importantly to improve the length and quality of life.

In the second definition, common sense, sagacity, and judgment are mentioned. Sagacity is defined as "keen intelligence; shrewdness." Knowledge of lasting truths (from the first definition) leads to common sense and good judgment. Suturing a wound that is contaminated will result in an infection. That was true for the first human that trod this earth, and will be true for the last. Any fool with a needle and thread can sew a wound shut. A wise doctor (and patient) realizes that the goal is not to close the wound, but to speed healing and minimize scarring.

Medical Wisdom

The quote from Thoreau is very applicable. When a person is seriously ill, desperate measures are often considered. Sometimes desperate measures will be suggested by doctors, but usually not. Patients (lacking medical wisdom) are most often the ones who seek and often employ desperate solutions. One desperate "solution," which arises from a lack of medical wisdom, is to deny there is a problem. We will discuss some of these desperate measures in this book, and you will acquire the wisdom to avoid such errors in judgment.

That leaves the third definition. Learning and erudition (defined as deep and extensive learning) is a form of wisdom, but only to the extent that it implies the first two definitions. The learning must result in an understanding and ability to apply that which is true, right, and lasting (first definition) in order to result in the common sense and judgment of the second definition.

Modern medicine is becoming increasingly complex…or is it really? Certainly the average person would agree that modern (scientific, Western) medicine is complicated and difficult to understand, but I argue that medicine has actually become, and continues to become, simpler. It is clear to me, as a teacher of emergency medicine, that when a medical concept is complete, accurate, and well understood, it is easy to teach and easily mastered. When a concept is incomplete, inaccurate, or less than well understood, it is very difficult to teach and impossible to learn. As medical science continues to make progress, more concepts become complete and accurate.

This morning I called a used bookstore to ask for directions. The first person I spoke to had a very difficult time telling me how to get there. I was running out of space on my notepad and becoming increasingly worried that I had misunderstood a few street names. Finally I asked for the address, thinking I would use "MapQuest" to look up the directions online. The employee didn't know the address! As it

Introduction

turned out, she had just started at the bookstore; when she handed the phone to a more experienced worker, that person gave me the directions in one sentence, which I easily understood, which made sense, and which I was able to remember without writing down! A medical concept, when complete and accurate, can be easily remembered, is easily taught, and can be built upon.

I have spent over fifteen years teaching these concepts to medical students, resident physicians, and patients. I have carefully considered everything I have been taught, and gone on to teach, while remaining critical. I know medicine "backward and forward" and can make it simple and real for you.

The field of medicine today is rapidly changing. Doctors have less time to spend with their patients, medical care is more costly, and a patient is less likely to receive medical care in a prompt manner. In the Pacific Northwest, the average wait to see an emergency physician last year was four hours and twenty-three minutes. Since "time is money," the cost of medical care is very high indeed! The health-care debate is an interesting one, but regardless of which direction we take as a country, knowing medicine will be very useful to you and will better enable you to control your destiny. This book will also help you when a loved one is ill.

The goal of this book is to help you become an educated (wise) consumer of medical care. I want you to know when something the doctor says makes sense. If something your doctor says doesn't make sense to you, I want you to have the foundation of knowledge required to ask the right questions.

Many of the patients I see in the ER do not need to be there. I am certainly glad to help them, but they could have easily avoided the time and expense if they'd had more medical wisdom.

In today's world patients need to be able to take an active part in their medical treatment. A doctor offers many options, and knowledge is required to make a good decision. Often your doctor would like to spend the hours it would take to teach you what you need to know to make a good decision, but he or she is only allowed fifteen minutes. In the ER, patients cannot make appointments, so I don't have the "fifteen-minute" problem that many primary-care physicians have. During our busy hours, however, we may have a dozen patients in the waiting room and all of our beds occupied by patients. At those busy times, I feel a great deal of pressure to work as fast as possible. During the small hours of the morning, the ER is not as busy, and I can sometimes take all the time I need. Being able to spend time with a patient is a luxury these days, and while it is gratifying, it makes me realize that complete medical care is not possible when I have to move quickly. My busy days help me understand the problem the office-based doctor faces when only fifteen minutes are allowed per patient.

There is no way I can teach you everything about medicine (I don't know everything there is to know—nobody does), but I can teach you the core concepts—concepts that have not changed and will not change until the human organism evolves beyond the flesh. In this book I do not intend to cover every possible medical problem, but I will cover the common problems within each area, as well as those less common problems that help to demonstrate important medical concepts.

Knowing the core concepts of human medicine will allow you to sort through new information intelligently. These days, a huge amount of medical information is available via the Internet, TV, books, and radio. Some of the information is accurate and good, but some is ridiculously (and harmfully) untrue.

My own mother died of colon cancer partially as a result of misinformation. She had heard that there were "thirty pounds of solid waste" in the average person's colon. I have heard such statements on the radio as well, and since my mother's death, they make me wince with pain. The truth: there is no stored waste! When a doctor orders a "barium enema," and the contrast (the liquid the X-ray cannot pass through to highlight the colon's interior) is placed, the entire colon can be visualized on an X-ray within minutes. There is nowhere for "stored solid waste" to hide. There are a few rare conditions of decreased colonic tone and transit, but over 99 percent of people have no "stored waste" at all. My mother spent many months trying to "clean out" and "decontaminate" the colon, when her feelings of fullness and her stool caliber change were actually caused by a slowly growing cancer.

My mother was highly educated in the areas of law and finance. She was a very intelligent woman. What she lacked was the medical wisdom required to recognize dangerous false information. Combined with the natural human tendency to ignore evil (disease in this case, which is a great evil), which we call denial, this lack of wisdom resulted in her untimely death. I have vowed to prevent as many others as possible from falling into that trap. The core medical concepts you will learn in this book will help you to recognize misinformation and to make better medical decisions for yourself and the ones you love.

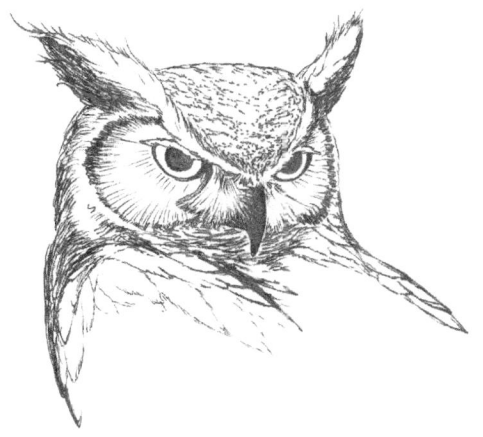

How the "System" of Modern Medicine Works

Medicine is a Science of Uncertainty, and an Art of Probability.

— ***Dr. William Osler***

A better title might be "the systematic approach to how we diagnose and treat disease in the modern world today." That is a bit long, though.

Much of what I tell you in this book is based on one of the most fundamental care-delivery units the country possesses: the emergency department (ED). My specialty is emergency medicine.

Medical Wisdom

Older patients I care for in the ED sometimes ask things like, "So what sort of specialty are you planning to go into when you are done here?" This was a good question forty years ago, because most doctors working in the ED were either very early in their careers or trying to start their practices. These doctors often were "doing some shifts" in the ER to make money on the side. Starting in the early 1970s, residency training in emergency medicine became available, and it was quickly realized that a serious need existed for trained emergency specialists. The specialty of emergency medicine is still growing, and the demand is still growing.

If you go to a "small-town ER" you may still see a doctor whose specialty is not emergency medicine. Trained emergency physicians are still in short supply, and most of them tend to work in the busier ERs, which both pay better and are more demanding of their skills.

When you first walk into the ER waiting room, you will generally go to the registration desk. You will be asked briefly about your problem. Just saying "headache" is enough at this stage, since you will have multiple chances to elaborate later. You will be asked for identification. The next step is called "triage" (pronounced tree-ahje), which means "sorting." There is usually a designated triage room, but if not, you may be taken straight to an examining room. Sometimes there is a triage nurse, and sometimes the nurse you will have for the remainder of your visit will do your triage. The triage nurse will ask you about your problem and gather some basic information. Your vital signs will be taken, and you will be classified into a category, or "triage level." If you are considered to be "stable" and there are no or few beds/rooms available, you may need to wait at this stage. If the problem is serious and has the potential to worsen, you will usually be taken straight to a room.

How the "System" of Modern Medicine Works

If more than one patient is waiting to be seen, I will look at the triage categories and pick the person in the highest category to see first. If two patients in the same category are waiting, I will see them in order of arrival. The downside of this system, from the perspective of a waiting patient, is that you may be next in line, but if an ambulance rolls in with a more seriously ill patient, you will be "bumped." This can happen again and again. If your doctor is the only one working, and a very sick patient comes in, he or she may be completely occupied with that patient. It may be minutes or even hours, before you will be seen. From the perspective of the very ill patient, of course, this system is a godsend.

If you go to a large teaching hospital, such as a university-affiliated facility, you will likely see more than one doctor during your ER visit. First, you might be seen by a medical student. The medical student should have a name tag announcing that status, and it is usually a different color than the doctor's tag. After the medical student, you may be seen by an intern (first-year resident) or a resident. If you are very ill, everyone may converge on you at the same time, including a nurse or two and possibly a tech and, if needed, a respiratory therapist. As you can see, the room can get crowded pretty fast! If the problem is stable and routine, the attending physician (professor) will see you last, after he hears a presentation from either the medical student or resident. The attending's job is both to ensure that all care at the teaching hospital is of the highest level and to teach the less-experienced physicians how to give that care.

New interns and medical students arrive in July, and the nurses will talk about that month in hushed tones. The attendings who work in July stay on their feet, and some of the older professors I knew always seemed to take July for vacation.

You may also be seen by a "midlevel provider." There are physician's assistants (PAs) and nurse practitioners (NPs). Both are similar in what they do. You may hear them referred to as "physician extenders." The training required for PAs and NPs is far less than that required for physicians, and some degree of physician supervision is legally required in most, if not all, situations. There are many times in the ER where an experienced midlevel provider can do an excellent job. Laceration repair, for example, can take a lot of time and requires a physician to wear sterile gloves and not leave the bedside. In a busy ER with many other patients, this can be a problem. A good midlevel can do an excellent and relaxed job of laceration repair, freeing up the physician to both supervise and see other patients. The increase in midlevel providers is partially driven by economics.

Your Doctor the Detective

When your doctor speaks to you he/she will be following an "investigative procedure" that has been instilled into the very core by years of teaching and discipline. Your doctor can follow this series of investigative steps, and will do so, without thinking. Your doctor can adhere to these steps even when half asleep, and completely exhausted. In fact, every doctor currently in practice has been subjected to much duress, sleeplessness, and tests of endurance. As an intern I often slept only every other night for months at a time. Laws have recently been passed that restrict the number of hours that an intern can work in a given week, but during internship and residency weeks with over a hundred hours of duty were not unusual. The "investigative procedure" is designed to reduce error and omission, even in the most difficult and stressful circumstances. If you understand this investigative procedure, you will be able to help your doctor do the best job possible. The investigation begins with the history, and ends with the diagnosis and treatment plan.

How the "System" of Modern Medicine Works

Your doctor will begin with the "history." We are taught to begin by asking an open ended question such as; "So what brought you to the ER today." We are then encouraged to listen without asking further questions for at least a few minutes. This listening part is hard to do, since the urge to ask pointed questions is great, and often overwhelming. Some of the history may have already been taken by the nurse, but be patient if your doctor confirms some of these points. The history includes not only the current problem, but past medical history, past surgical history, allergies and more.

Next your doctor will review your vital signs, and any other objective data that is available. The doctor will consider if there will be other information needed at this point, and may order some laboratory tests or X-rays if ordering at this point will save time and help you if there is a chance of rapid worsening.

The physical exam is the next step. On an initial office visit your personal physician will perform a thorough (comprehensive) physical exam. During the following visits the exam will be briefer and more focused. In the ED your exam will generally be focused around the reason for your visit. If you have an ankle injury, I will examine the foot, ankle and knee. I will observe, palpate, and test function. I will ask if there are other injuries or problems, and if you fell will examine the other injuries as well. If the problem is more complex, such as shortness of breath, a much more thorough examination will be needed.

At this point tests will be ordered if needed to complete the information required to make accurate decisions. Treatment will continue at this point as well.

The final step is the assessment and plan. The subjective (history) and objective (exam, labs, etc.) information is integrated and a number of diagnoses are considered. The list of possible diagnoses is known as the "differential diagnosis." A simple problem will have a short list of possibilities, and a more complex problem a longer list. If the diagnosis upon which treatment is based is correct, improvement should occur. If improvement does not occur as expected, the information is reconsidered and another direction of treatment starts. "Follow up," and ongoing care is arranged.

Helping your doctor to gather an adequate history, and mentioning anything you feel is notable during the physical exam, will improve the odds that the right diagnosis is found, and proper treatment initiated.

Convention vs. Common Sense

Sometimes in modern medicine, "conventional practice" conflicts with "common sense." In these situations, I will give examples so you can come away with the common sense—and smile at what the doctor tells you!

Much of what we do in medical practice is based on percentages. You will see that very little in medicine is "black and white." I can usually give a good percentage estimate of outcomes, based on my training and experience with a problem, but the human system is too complex and constantly changing to be predicted with absolute accuracy.

Doctors in the civilian United States need to "play it safer" than in some other places. This is partially to protect the patient and partially to protect themselves. Doctors are concerned about lawsuits, of course, as they are stressful, difficult, usually insulting, and potentially costly. There is also the ironic fact that there has never been an association between quality of medical care and chance of a lawsuit! What this basically means to a doctor is that when it comes to lawsuits, it "just doesn't matter; you're going to get sued sooner or later." I have heard that the average is every six years nowadays.

How the "System" of Modern Medicine Works

Would decreasing the cost of lawsuits decrease the cost of medical care? Certainly it would, but possibly not as much as people tend to think. Doctors are much more worried about doing the right thing for their patients than they are about lawsuits. I never order a test to reduce risk of a lawsuit; I order only those tests that will benefit my patients. Many people blame the increased cost of health care on "defensive medicine," but the truth is, we are defending our patients much more often than ourselves. If there is less risk of big lawsuits, then the cost of malpractice insurance would decrease, saving doctors and hospitals money. Such a change is known as "tort reform" and does save some money, but not enough to make a huge difference.

Medical care in the United States is expensive for several reasons. First, it is very, very good and technically advanced. If you don't have an MRI scanner, for example, the cost of MRI scans suddenly drops to zero! You will also not detect subtle problems, such as a minor brain injury, early cancer while it is still curable, and multiple sclerosis. Because these serious problems are not detected, yet more money is saved by not having to treat them!

Second, it is a big system with a lot of complex infrastructure and redundancy. When I see a patient in the ER, my charges as a physician are only about twenty percent of the total bill for the visit, and often they are less than that. The facility charges and other costs make up the rest. The care system in which I work is excellent, and we are set up to take emergency care of any medical problem that exists. When someone with a minor problem comes in, we certainly take care of them in an efficient and excellent manner, but the cost of being "ready for anything" makes it more expensive.

Third, medical care is expensive in the United States because most people don't pay for it directly. I am familiar with three recent bills for laceration repair in the ER. In each case the lacerations were less than one inch (2.5 cm.) in length, and located on a finger. The bills varied from 1572.00 to 2100.00 USD. Of that bill, the patients were responsible for between zero and one hundred dollars. As a physician, my share of the bill was less than 300.00 in each instance. I am sure that if patients were actually required to pay the whole bill, there would be a stronger push for decreasing cost.

Thirty Seventh in the world...hmm, I have a bridge to sell you!

Don't buy in to the "United States is ranked thirty-seventh in the world" blanket statement you have heard. That rumor was started by the 2000 World Health Organization ranking. The number is usually quoted by people who have never seen the report. If they took the time to look at the report, they would see that thirty-seventh is in a particular category. The category is a complex and somewhat subjective one involving "how good we do with health care for the amount of money spent." It is an "efficiency" ranking, in other words. Since we (fortunately or unfortunately, depending on whether you are currently ill or well) ranked number one in the amount spent per person, we started out with a big disadvantage in that category! We ranked number one in several categories that you will no doubt consider more important than efficiency if you are ill.

Only someone with their "head in a gopher burrow" could have believed that the United States ranked thirty-seventh in health care. Where do people who want the best medical care come? To the United States, of course! Where do the vast majority of advancements in medical care come from? The United States, of course!

How the "System" of Modern Medicine Works

Health care in this country is the best in the world. It is, however, the most expensive for the people. I suppose we "get what we pay for." More efficiency is needed, though, and some of that efficiency can start with the consumer. This book will help you to be more efficient when it comes to health care.

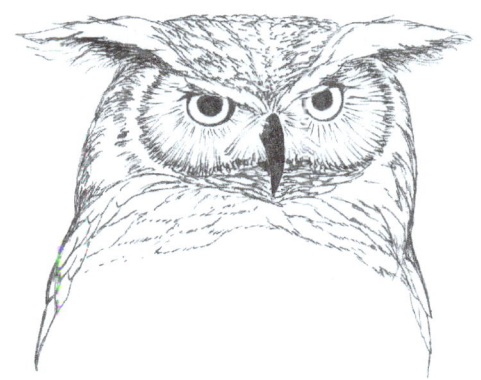

How to Use this Book

This book is intended to be read from cover to cover initially and then to be kept as a reference. The various chapters will combine, as if they were pieces of a puzzle, to create a "core" of medical knowledge. If you have had a serious medical problem, or are currently dealing with a medical problem, then there is nothing wrong with finding that problem in the table of contents, and reading that chapter first. Realize that the information in this book builds to some extent upon the earlier information. If you return to that chapter of interest after finishing the book, you will find that it means more to you than before.

Keeping this book concise has been my most difficult challenge. Avoiding repetition has been essential. For example, many of the concepts of abdominal pain also apply to pelvic pain. If you read only the pelvic pain section, you will miss some important points. If you have read the entire book, and then later develop pelvic pain, a review of the pelvic pain section should suffice. Keeping the book among your references will allow you to review specific chapters as you encounter medical problems and injuries.

If you have an ongoing medical problem, you likely have learned a lot about it from your multifaceted experience. Your depth of knowledge about that particular problem may be great. This book will help you to sort through what you have learned, and if a concept you have held as a stable piece of data suddenly doesn't make sense anymore, don't be surprised!

Some knowledge of anatomy (how it's built) and physiology (how it works) is often needed to understand pathophysiology (how it breaks down). Depending on your educational background, some of this information may be review for you. Many highly intelligent and thoroughly educated people have very little biological and medical knowledge. In today's world that is a deficit that needs to be remedied!

In this book I use the terms ER (emergency room) and ED (emergency department) interchangeably. In the olden days, there was often a single room, known as the emergency room. Now most ERs are large departments with many rooms, triage (sorting of patients) areas, registration, nursing stations, and offices. Most emergency physicians prefer "emergency department" over "emergency room," but sometimes "ER" just sounds better.

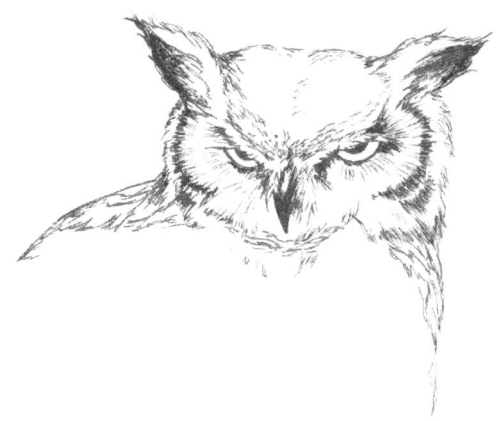

Chapter 1
Abdominal Pain

The first, and most important, thing to discover in the evaluation of a patient with abdominal pain is whether or not the abdomen is tender. A tender abdomen is a surgical problem, until proven otherwise.

—Dr. Jeffrey Ponsky, surgeon and professor,
Case Western Reserve University, Cleveland, OH

Certainly this is a "meaty" subject with which to begin, but an important one. In most years, abdominal pain competes with chest pain as the commonest cause of visits to the ER. Abdominal pain is a potentially dangerous and often complex problem.

Abdominal pain can be classified as "acute" or "chronic." Your doctor will initially attempt to determine if this pain is new to you, or if you have had it on and off for months or years. Though there are serious abdominal problems of long duration, most of the potentially life-threatening problems will be "acute." If you have significant abdominal pain that you have not previously experienced, then a prompt call to your doctor and/or a visit to the ER is a good idea.

Associated symptoms are important to note. Other concerning features, such as fever, persistent vomiting, and dehydration, when accompanied by abdominal pain, should prompt you to seek medical help. A rapid heart rate (tachycardia), fever, and decreased blood pressure are particularly concerning when preceded and/or accompanied by abdominal pain. Fever in the presence of significant and persistent abdominal pain is almost always a serious problem and often will require hospitalization and surgery.

Where is the Pain?

Abdominal pain can sometimes be felt clearly and localized precisely, and sometimes it is vague and poorly localized. These two types of pain are known as "peritoneal pain" and "visceral pain." The peritoneum is the layer of tissue that surrounds the abdominal contents, and it is very sensitive. The average young person has never felt peritoneal abdominal pain. Almost everyone has felt visceral abdominal pain, a variety of which often occurs before vomiting or diarrhea. When asked, "Where is the pain?" the patient with visceral abdominal pain will often point to the midabdomen or umbilicus, or wave across the entire abdomen. Peritoneal abdominal pain can be diffuse, but only if the entire inside of the abdomen is involved. When a specific part of the peritoneum is injured or irritated, the patient can point to the spot

Chapter 1 Abdominal Pain

A Classic Case of Appendicitis

Several months ago I diagnosed a classic (the way they describe it in medical school), but unfortunately late-presenting, case of appendicitis. Appendicitis is an excellent demonstration of the progression of a visceral (poorly localized) abdominal pain to a peritoneal (well localized) one.

The patient, a thirty-one-year-old elementary schoolteacher named Bill, first developed pain three days before arriving in the emergency department. Initially the pain was "a dull ache" across the central abdomen, accompanied by mild loss of appetite and nausea. Bill tried some medicine for nausea, which helped a little, but the pain continued. He also tried some Motrin, which he promptly vomited. Toward the end of the first day, he noticed that the pain was becoming worse in the right lower abdomen and that it hurt with walking and moving. Bill decided to see if he could "sleep it off." He admitted that he worried it might be appendicitis, but he was not enthusiastic about the idea of surgery, and he had "heard of appendicitis going away by itself." Bill lived alone, and there was no one to encourage him to seek help. He slept poorly, and by four in the morning, the intermittent warm feelings had become a sustained fever. He then managed to drive, with great pain, to the ER.

When I first saw him, he looked ill. His temperature was elevated, his heart rate fast, and he was sweaty (diaphoretic) and pale. He looked dehydrated and though he was thirsty, was nauseated and had not been able to drink. While I examined him, I asked the nurse to prepare to start an IV and to give a two-liter normal saline bolus followed by a rate of 200 milliliters per hour. At this time I also ordered antibiotics (to be given IV). On abdominal exam, Bill's abdomen was very tender, and while it was most tender in the right lower "quadrant," there was also some diffuse pain. Lightly shaking the bed caused pain, and Bill said that "every bump on the drive was painful."

I called the surgeon immediately, and given the clear-cut case, no additional testing was needed. Within two hours, Bill's appendix was removed. The appendix had just ruptured, and the surgery and Bill's recovery were more difficult than if he had come to the ER earlier.

Note that Bill's pain started as a dull ache that he could not easily localize. At that time the appendix, which is a vestigial (remnant, no longer needed) tubular structure attached to the large intestine near the junction of the large and small intestines, had become obstructed and was becoming swollen. The bowel is sensitive to stretch, and the aching, diffuse pain of a stretched bowel is familiar to all of us. As the inflammation continued, the appendix began to irritate the peritoneum, and Bill was then able to point to the right lower abdomen.

At some point the appendix ruptured, releasing the pressure. At this point the pain would typically decrease, but the infection within the appendix would have been released into the abdomen, causing the more serious (life-threatening) problem of peritonitis. As the infection spread throughout the abdomen, the pain increased once again and became more diffuse.

After rupture, fever and diffuse pain/chills and a very ill appearance are typical. Palpation of the abdomen after rupture will demonstrate severe, diffuse tenderness, and the patient will involuntarily tense the abdominal muscles, causing a "rigid" abdomen. There are rare reports of recurrent appendicitis, and certainly it is conceivable that an obstruction of the appendix could be relieved spontaneously, but betting on the spontaneous resolution of appendicitis is a losing game.

Most medical professionals would call Bill's delay "denial." There is a strong tendency in humans to deny that a serious problem is present, and we should all be aware of that tendency, in both ourselves and our loved ones.

Chapter 1 Abdominal Pain

Although localizing the pain can be difficult at times, the location of pain, as well as the progression and radiation (where the pain extends to/moves to) can be important. The pain of appendicitis, though beginning diffusely, should move to the right lower abdomen as the inflammation affects the peritoneal tissue.

Diverticulitis

Diverticulitis is a process similar to appendicitis in some ways. A diverticulum is a small out-pouching of a hollow structure. Diverticula of the large bowel are commoner in older people and can become blocked off, with the same resultant inflammation and rupture that occurs in acute appendicitis.

In diverticulitis the problem is better confined, and a localized problem occurs, rather than an infection of the entire abdomen. Diverticulitis most often occurs in the left lower abdomen (the descending colon), and the pain is generally well localized, as the peritoneum is involved earlier in the process. Antibiotics are often effective in controlling diverticulitis, but if there is a fever, elevated white blood cell count, or palpable swelling, a CT scan (see the "X-Ray and Radiology" chapter) will often be done, and if there is an abscess (walled off area of infection), a surgeon should be consulted.

Your doctor will ask if there are things that make the abdominal pain worse or better. In the case of appendicitis that has progressed and other forms of peritonitis, moving suddenly or walking often makes the pain worse, and remaining still will give some relief. In stomach, esophageal, and duodenal (the first part of the small intestine) pain, eating will affect the pain. Eating and drinking irritating liquids, such as alcohol-containing drinks, worsens pain of the esophagus and stomach. Eating can decrease the pain of a duodenal ulcer, presumably by mixing food with the stomach acid and thus decreasing the acidity of the material to which the ulcer, located at a point just after the stomach (duodenum), is exposed. Sometimes this effect is so pronounced that a person with a duodenal ulcer will gain a substantial amount of weight.

When the Bowel "Telescopes" and Other Intestinal Obstructions

The small and large intestines can occasionally become completely or partially obstructed. When this occurs, an intermittent, cramping pain (which is difficult to precisely localize) is typical.

In children, the four primary ways this can happen are pyloric stenosis, midgut volvulus (twisting of the bowel, which also can happen in adults), intussusception, and constipation.

Pyloric stenosis is commonest in the one- to three-month-old child. The pylorus is the valve between the stomach and the duodenum, and in pyloric stenosis this valve becomes too thickened, decreasing flow out of the stomach. Vomiting of undigested milk or formula that progressively worsens, becoming "projectile," is typical. Pyloric stenosis is commoner in males than females, and a "six week old first born male" is the "classic" case. Progressive dehydration and weight loss can occur. If this problem is suspected, calling the pediatrician promptly is a good idea. Ultrasound is often used to diagnose pyloric stenosis, and surgery to correct the problem may be needed.

Midgut volvulus results from a twisting of the bowel. Intermittent severe pain and vomiting are typical, and the vomiting is often bilious (bitter and yellow colored). Midgut volvulus occurs more frequently in infants, but can occur at any age range. Plain X-rays will be done initially, and immediate surgical consultation is needed. Intussusception occurs most frequently in the five-month to three-year age range, though it should be considered in all children younger than six years.

Intussusception occurs when the bowel "telescopes" or involutes upon itself, causing obstruction. Intermittent, severe cramping pain is typical, with vomiting usually; the classic case is of a toddler who plays unconcerned between short episodes of loud crying and distress. Bloody stool may occur, but this is not reliably present. If intussusception is suspected, a prompt trip to the ER is indicated, and you should tell the doctor that you came because you were worried about intussusception. Don't worry if you can't pronounce it; your doctor may just nod, rather than repeating it, for the same reason! The reason you need to tell your doctor (as with appendicitis), is that intussusception is easy for even a good doctor to miss. A plain X-ray will be done initially, and if the problem is still suspected, a barium enema is usually diagnostic and often curative.

Bowel obstruction and partial bowel obstruction in adults are often associated with postsurgical scarring and adhesions (scar tissue connecting/pulling on or restricting the movement of some structures not normally connected). Bowel obstruction in adults also causes intermittent, severe pain, vomiting, and distension. The degree of distension is frequently greater than in children. The amount of vomiting that occurs with complete obstruction is often impressive and will exceed several liters a day. Surgery is often needed to relieve the obstruction, though placement of a "nasogastric" tube, rehydration, and pain control will often allow the obstruction to ease or resolve.

I have certainly treated hundreds of cases of constipation in the emergency department. Constipation will often cause the poorly localized (visceral), intermittent cramping pain characteristic of bowel obstruction. In its severest form, constipation can cause obstruction and at that point is called "obstipation."

In children constipation tends to occur at specific ages. Congenital gastrointestinal defects, depending on the specific problem, become apparent early. Hopefully the pediatrician notes an "imperforate anus" early! Many new parents can be reassured that "three bowel movements a week to three a day is normal." When the child begins to take solid foods (currently recommended to be introduced gradually, starting at six months) the solidity and frequency of bowel movements change; sometimes this change begins as a period of decreased frequency as the bowel adapts to the greater amount of solid matter. During the potty training period, there are frequently problems with constipation, and when school becomes more demanding, constipation can occur as trips to the bathroom are delayed. (At least one of the students in my medical school class had this problem, and several of us felt it was our responsibility to help him. Things didn't go all that well…but he did survive!)

The Ping-Pong Ball Principle

To understand constipation, it is important to understand how the colon and rectum work. The primary purpose of the colon (a.k.a. large intestine) is to remove water from the body's solid waste. As the stool becomes solid, it is moved into the rectum, and water continues to be removed. When the rectum is distended, the stretching is felt as a fullness and an urge to have a bowel movement. If the urge is ignored, it will likely pass, but the absorption of water from the stool will continue. In this way the problem is perpetuated.

The urge to have a bowel movement is known as "tenesmus." Tenesmus is also caused by the stretching of a swollen hemorrhoid (swollen vein near the rectum), and a person with a hemorrhoid will feel as if the rectum is still distended. Continued straining will be nonproductive and causes further swelling of the hemorrhoid, which in turn causes more tenesmus. By these two mechanisms, the hemorrhoid is worsened. Opiate pain medications such as codeine can cause slowing of bowel transit (more time to absorb water) and thus should be taken with stool softeners.

I have asked numerous patients if they understand how fiber-containing products such as Metamucil and Citrucel could possibly help constipation, and in general they don't understand. Often a patient will try one dose, see no result, and stop. The key to these products is daily use. In medical school we used to joke about the "ping-pong ball principle," wherein the brain could only hold so much information—like a roll of toilet paper and a bunch of ping-pong balls. When a person keeps putting more and more ping-pong balls in one side, eventually a ball will fall out the other side each time a new one is put in. We all agreed that the brain is not that simple, but occasionally it was a good excuse to ignore something that didn't make sense! The bowel is essentially a tube of limited capacity, and if a good amount of non-absorbable fiber goes in one side each day, it will come out the other. Each day is the key, and if some comes out each day, the rectum will not have extra time to dry and harden the stool excessively.

In general, people have more problems with constipation as they get older. This is primarily caused by decreased muscle tone combined with drier tissues overall. If the bowel is not strong enough to push the stool along, the temptation to use enemas and laxative arises. If these are used repeatedly, the bowel's tone and strength will continue to decrease, resulting in further constipation. Laxatives should therefore be used with caution. If there is a serious blockage below, it needs to be cleared by enema, suppository, or manually before oral laxatives should be given.

More Causes of Abdominal Pain

"Gastroenteritis," an infection of the stomach and intestines, and "food poisoning" are occasionally tough to distinguish from the more serious causes of pain. Usually in gastroenteritis, the vomiting and diarrhea precedes the pain. (We will discuss gastroenteritis more in the "Nausea, Vomiting, and Diarrhea" chapter.) Pain is generally the secondary problem in gastroenteritis, and it is mild. If pain is the primary problem, or if the abdomen is tender, a more serious cause should be considered.

Abdominal pain can come from the urinary tract (kidneys, ureters, and bladder). Pain in the "flank" area is typical with kidney stones and kidney infection. Bladder pain from infection is often described as "burning," radiating to the urethra or flanks, and is often worst with and after urination. Kidney-stone pain is sharp, intermittently more severe, and not much affected by movement (see the "Urinary Problems" chapter).

In older patients and those with known vascular problems, abdominal pain can be caused by bowel ischemia or blood-vessel failure (decreased blood flow/dissection). (See also the "Chest Pain" chapter and the sections on lower extremity pain in the "Extremity Pain" chapters.)

A significant cause of serious abdominal pain in the older population is the gallbladder. "Biliary colic" is the phrase used to describe the pain that occurs as the gallbladder (a relatively small structure attached to the liver that stores bile, releasing it as needed into the duodenum) contracts against some sort of obstruction. The term "biliary colic" is a misnomer, as the pain is not an intermittent (colicky) pain, but a persistent one. The gallbladder is located in the right upper abdomen, and the pain is usually somewhat vague, often generalized across the upper abdomen or radiating toward the sternum or back. Older people in general seem to become more tolerant of pain and will sometimes minimize the pain of recurrent biliary colic.

The bile stored in the gallbladder is similar in color and has the same oily/soapy feel as yellow dishwashing detergent. Bile also serves the same purpose as dishwashing detergent. When trying to wash the frying pan after cooking some hamburgers, the water seems to have no effect on the greasy residue. A few drops of soap, however, and the grease is broken up into smaller parts, which can be washed away. When a person eats fatty foods, the gallbladder contracts, releasing bile. Bile "emulsifies" (breaks down into smaller particles) the fat, which allows it to be absorbed. Cholelithiasis (gallstones) can cause a blockage of the gallbladder where it drains into the bowel. A gallstone can also block the drainage from both the gallbladder and pancreas, and these blockages, if not relieved, can be life threatening.

Chapter 1 Abdominal Pain

When Gallbladder Pain Becomes Serious

Often an older person has been living with the pain of gallstones for many years and has learned to deal with the pain by avoiding fatty foods and suffering through the pain when it occurs. This was the case with Charlene, who at eighty years of age had her usual full day, which started with walking her dog the mile to Starbucks for her morning coffee. She then ate a banana, did some gardening work, and played golf with friends. Though she had learned to avoid fatty foods, she had a large dinner at a friend's house that included steak. Shortly after dinner she had her "gallbladder pain." Hoping it would go away, she went to bed. The pain persisted and made it hard to sleep. She vomited several times, but this didn't seem to help. By morning the pain had worsened; she had vomited several more times during the night and decided to stay in bed. Her husband of almost sixty years was very concerned and called her doctor, who recommended she go to the ER.

When she arrived in the ER, Charlene looked pale, and though she walked in, it was hard to picture her walking nine holes of golf less than a day earlier. She appeared dehydrated, insisted on holding an emesis basin during the examination, and though she asked for something to drink, refused to drink the water her husband offered her. On examination her abdomen was very tender, and she was reluctant to have me feel the upper abdomen and especially the right upper quadrant. The pain was clearly worse around the gallbladder. She mentioned that she had had this same sort of pain for years, but it had never lasted this long. Charlene felt better after some pain medication and IV rehydration. Her blood showed elevated liver and pancreatic enzymes and an elevated white blood cell count, as well (see "The Medical Laboratory" chapter). The ultrasound showed a gallstone obstructing the common duct through which the gallbladder and pancreas both excrete their products into the duodenum. Gallstone pancreatitis is a serious problem, and despite optimal treatment, Charlene got much worse before she improved. She spent several weeks in the intensive care unit, had her gallbladder removed after antibiotics and endoscopic stone removal had relieved the inflammation, and is back on the golf course. Those who choose to live with gallstones, rather than having surgery, should be aware of the signs of gallstone-associated problems.

If you are female and have lower abdominal pain, expect a pregnancy test and a pelvic exam. Pregnancy is something your doctor cannot afford to miss, and patients claiming in the emergency department that there is "absolutely no chance of pregnancy" are found to be pregnant up to 20 percent of the time! (Patients who said there was a "very small chance" were pregnant less than 10 percent of the time!) Significant abdominal pain early in pregnancy can be caused by an ectopic (in the wrong place) pregnancy (see the "Pregnancy-related Problems" chapter). The pelvic exam will look for external causes of pain, such as rashes, for signs of infection or injury, and for cancer/tumor (see the discussion of pelvic pain in the "Trauma" chapter).

If you arrive in the emergency department with significant acute abdominal pain, you should expect rapid assessment, called "triage." Vital signs will be taken initially, and if these are abnormal, you should be seen and treated as soon as possible. Medicine for pain and nausea should be given early in your stay.

Until about fifteen years ago, many surgeons felt that pain medicine should not be given to patients with abdominal pain. They argued that the pain medicine would make their examination of the abdomen less reliable. As the quote by Dr. Ponsky at the start of this chapter demonstrates, the abdominal exam is very important and more important than laboratory tests in many cases. It is the rare surgeon nowadays who will withhold pain medication, and most realize that the effect on the examination is minimal, while the ben-efit to the patient is significant. If someone withholds pain medica-tion, stating that "the surgeon will need to see you/your loved one first," suggesting a short-acting pain medication such as Fentanyl is a good idea.

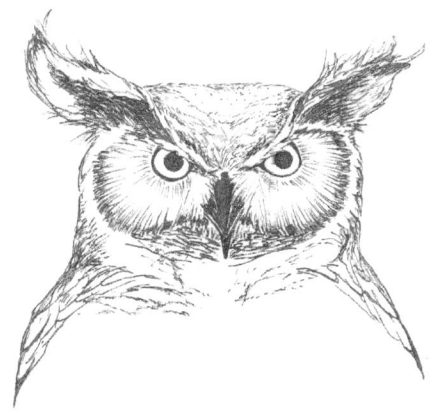

Chapter 2
Anemia

And so it was that later,
As the Miller told his tale.
That at first her face just ghostly,
Turned a whiter shade of pale.
—Lyrics from Procol Harem's "A Lighter Shade of Pale"

Anemia is the loss of blood or the failure to make the cellular part of the blood, resulting in blood that is too "thin." When a person loses blood faster than new blood cells can be made, the amount of red cells available to carry oxygen is decreased.

15

Medical Wisdom

The primary measure of anemia is the "hematocrit," which is the percentage of cells in the blood. In medical school, I learned how to use a centrifuge to "spin" blood down so that the cells would settle into an opaque layer and the serum would remain in a clear layer above. We would then measure the percentage of the total sample volume occupied by the cells (opaque lower layer), and that percentage was the hematocrit. Nowadays the computation of hematocrit is mostly done by a machine, which also describes the cells, both white and red. This description of the cells is known as the "differential." A normal hematocrit is between 35 percent and 50 percent. In other words, a bit less than half the mass of the blood is made up of cells, both red and white.

The primary function of red blood cells is to carry oxygen, and white blood cells are the body's defense system. The two primary categories of white blood cells are the lymphocytes and phagocytes. Lymphocytes secrete antibodies (b-cells) and activate defenses (t-cells). Phagocytes ingest and digest bacteria and other threats to the body. The system of defense is complex, and we will discuss it further in the following chapters.

When blood is suddenly lost, both serum and cells are lost. The volume of serum is easily replaced, and much of that volume is replaced within minutes. Fluid from within the cells and tissue move into the vascular space (bloodstream), and the blood volume is partially restored. After this has occurred, however, the hematocrit is initially reduced, as the cells have not been replaced. Blood is constantly being made, and if the loss of blood ceases, the hematocrit will be restored by cells manufactured within the bone marrow and released into the blood.

Anemia is sometimes recognized by a pale skin color or by changes in color of the nail beds or lips. I find the color of the inside of the eyelids to be most helpful, and if you turn out your lower eyelid and look at the color in the mirror, you will notice that (unless you are anemic) there is a nice pink/red color. When this pink/red color is lost, there is usually a substantial decrease in the hematocrit. Another sign of anemia can be shortness of breath, though this can be a late sign, especially in younger people.

Blood Lost vs. Blood Not Made

The causes of anemia are divided into two primary categories: anemia caused by blood loss and anemia caused by decreased manufacture of blood.

The commonest source of blood loss that is not noticed is the stool. A significant amount of blood can be lost in the stool without it being visible. A "hemocult" test is a screening test for invisible blood loss in which a small amount of stool is placed on a card and a drop of developer applied. Your doctor will perform this test after a rectal exam and may send you home with some cards to use over a period of days. Blood can also be lost in the urine without being obvious, and at times a woman's menses can be heavy enough to cause anemia.

Deficiency of iron, vitamin B-12, or folic acid can cause anemia. Anemia caused by low iron stores is characterized by smaller-than-usual red blood cells. Iron is needed to make blood cells because they contain hemoglobin, which is rich in iron. Vitamin B-12 deficiency anemia, also called "pernicious anemia," causes large, underdeveloped red blood cells to be produced. Folic acid deficiency also causes these large red cells. For this reason, these causes of anemia are known as megaloblastic. Folic acid is found in citrus fruit and green, leafy vegetables. A diet deficient in these, without supplementation, can result in megaloblastic anemia.

Vitamin B-12 deficiency anemia is sometimes found in strict vegetarians, as B-12 is found primarily in meats, eggs, and milk. Most commonly, B-12 deficiency is found because of a lack of "intrinsic factor." Intrinsic factor is made in the stomach and binds to B-12, allowing it to be absorbed in the intestine. Lack of intrinsic factor, and the resultant pernicious (deadly) anemia, was a potentially serious problem before B-12 shots were available.

Lower-than-expected levels of either platelets (a smaller blood product vital to forming blood clots) or white blood cells can also cause problems.

If you are found to have anemia or a low blood count, further testing will be needed to determine the cause.

Blood transfusion may be needed if the blood count is especially low, if there is continued bleeding and anticipated further bleeding, or if you are having symptoms as a result of the decreased level.

Pros and Cons of Transfusions

Blood transfusion is not without risks and should be carefully considered. Infection related to blood transfusion is less likely today than in earlier years since our screening has improved, but there is still a risk. One risk is a transfusion reaction, which is when transfused blood is recognized as "alien" by the body's immune system and is attacked. In the blood bank or laboratory, the blood is tested and the recipient's blood type and antigens are determined. Blood of that same type is chosen as potentially compatible, and that blood is then mixed with some of the recipient's serum. If there is no clumping or adverse reaction, the match is considered good.

In a serious emergency, blood that is not cross matched can be transfused, and this blood can be either the same type as the recipient's (preferred) or if the recipient's type is not yet known, O negative (type O, Rh antigen negative).

A healthy young patient with a known source of bleeding that has been controlled can tolerate a hematocrit in the teens without danger. A frequent example of this scenario, and one in which transfusion is often not performed, is the young female who has had excessive bleeding as the result of a pregnancy-related problem.

Most physicians will recommend blood transfusion for a hematocrit below 20 percent. As more studies are done, it is becoming clearer that transfusion problems outweigh benefits if the hematocrit is between 25 percent and 30 percent. A blood transfusion is increasingly being viewed as an "organ transplant." This view makes sense: there appear to be some problems associated with transfusion that are not easily quantified but result in people not doing as well as expected afterward. In the "gray" area of 20–25 percent there is an increasing trend toward avoiding transfusion. The amount of blood needed varies, and the goal in general is to raise the percentage of cells (the hematocrit) to around 30 percent.

In deciding whether or not to transfuse it is most important to judge how well the person is handling the low blood level. Tolerance of activity is an important measure, and if the person's heart is working harder than usual while they are inactive, transfusion is often recommended. An elevated pulse rate would be expected, and this would be caused by the attempt to compensate for decreased oxygen delivery per liter of blood, by delivering more liters of blood.

Measuring the Pulse Rate

To measure a person's pulse rate per minute, count the pulse over a fifteen second period and multiply by four. There are three common places to feel the human pulse. As we go over this, be sure to find your own pulse at each location. The ability to measure your own heart rate will often be useful.

The first location to feel a pulse is the radial artery. To find the radial artery, feel on the soft (under) side of the wrist, on the thumb (radial) side about an inch toward the elbow from the wrist crease. Press hard enough to partially block the blood flow, and you should feel it easily. The radial pulse is a common place to check, but as the blood pressure drops, it will be one of the first to decrease in strength. We will discuss this in the "Trauma" chapter.

Medical Wisdom

The carotid pulse is strong, easy to find, and can be felt even if the blood pressure is low. To find the carotid pulse, take the index and long fingers of your right hand and lay them flat across the left side of your neck at the level of the "Adam's apple," known medically as the thyroid cartilage. Your thumb will be on the right side of the windpipe (trachea). Press in with the flattened fingers and you will feel the pulse. The pulse is easier to feel higher on the neck, than lower. The carotid pulse is a good one to check while you are on a treadmill, and is the one you will feel for if you examine an unconscious person.

The femoral pulse is harder to find on oneself than the others, because of the angle. To find the femoral pulse on another person, lay the flats of your fingers along the hip crease, and press hard enough to partially occlude the femoral artery.

Pulse rate and heart rate are the same in normal circumstances. We will discuss a heart problem called "atrial fibrillation" in the "Shortness of Breath" chapter that often causes unproductive heart beats that do not create a pulse. Feeling the heart itself through the chest wall is often possible. When I feel an irregular pulse, I often listen to the heart with my stethoscope while feeling the pulse to see if there are heartbeats that do not create a pulse.

If you are scheduled for an elective surgery, a good option is to donate some of your own blood, which can be used if needed. Artificial oxygen-transporting substances offer hope for the future, but currently there is no truly safe and effective blood substitute.

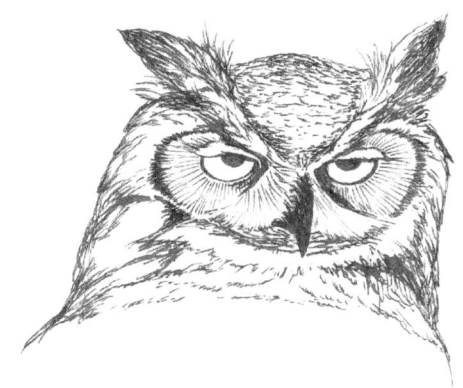

Chapter 3
Autoimmune Diseases

You can choose a ready guide in some celestial voice
if you choose not to decide, you still have made a choice
You can choose from phantom fears and kindness that can kill
I will choose a path that's clear
I will choose freewill

—Lyrics from the song "Freewill" by Rush

Sometimes the body's defense system attacks the body itself. There are more than eighty different diseases in which this is the case, and the results are highly varied.

Medical Wisdom

The first difficulty a patient with an autoimmune problem faces is getting diagnosed. The best bet is to see one's primary doctor initially, and then if needed see the specialist most closely related to the primary symptom. For example, if joint pain is the problem, a rheumatologist would be the specialist to see. Symptoms can be as vague as tiredness and aching muscles, and since the severity of the symptoms can vary over time, with spontaneous remissions frequently occurring, diagnosis is even more difficult.

Autoimmune diseases can affect multiple body systems, or the attack can be more localized, affecting a specific organ. Common autoimmune diseases affecting the whole body (systemic) include rheumatoid arthritis, lupus, and polymyalgia rheumatica. Attacks on a single organ include early onset diabetes, wherein the pancreas is attacked, and Graves' disease, in which the thyroid is attacked.

Leading a healthy lifestyle may not help. Since it is your own body causing the problem, optimizing your immunity with vitamins, exercise, and adequate sleep is not likely to decrease the symptoms.

A number of drugs can decrease the efficiency of a person's immune system, and these often help to decrease the symptoms. We will discuss these drugs again in the "Medications" chapter.

The "mildest" of this group of drugs is the "nonsteroidal anti-inflammatory drugs": aspirin, ibuprofen, naproxen, and many others. These drugs reduce pain and have a mild effect on the body's immune system.

The second type, corticosteroids, have a greater effect on the immune system, but their other hormonal effects cause problems if used on a long-term basis. Corticosteroids are definitely not the same as the performance-enhancing steroids we hear so much about on the news.

Chapter 3 Autoimmune Diseases

The third type of drugs used in autoimmune-disease treatment is the immunosuppressant agents. These drugs include Cytoxan and methotrexate. These powerful drugs act to blunt the body's immune system and should be monitored carefully for undesired side effects.

Sometimes the cause of an autoimmune exacerbation can be found, and lifestyle changes can help prevent recurrence.

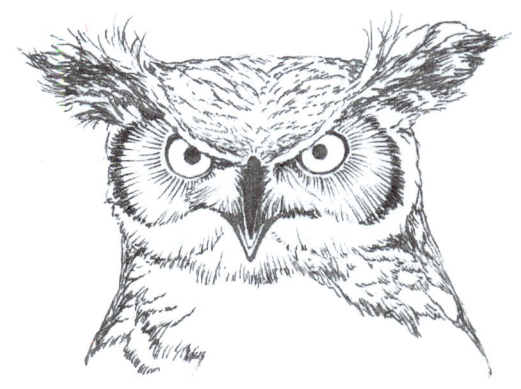

Chapter 4
Back Pain

"What a man needs in gardening is a cast-iron back, with a hinge in it."

—Charles Dudley Warner

Back pain is a common cause of emergency department visits. Rarely do I work a shift without seeing at least a few patients with back pain, and pain in the low back is the most common. Serious back pain requiring medical treatment and resulting in lost income is experienced by over half of adult Americans. Back pain also tends to be recurrent, and the majority of people who have had back pain will have recurrent pain.

The primary components of the back are bone, muscle, cartilage, and nerves. The vertebral bones are stacked in a column, separated by cushions of cartilage known as "discs." Each disc has a tough outer layer and a more fluid inner layer. The spinal cord is located behind the vertebral column and is protected by a "cage" of bone, which also helps to add to strength and stability. Between each level of the column, nerve roots emerge, providing sensation and function to different levels of the body. The nerves of the lumbar spine and sacrum go to the legs and genital area, while the nerves of the neck supply the arms. Muscles surround the spine, provide further support. The abdominal muscles and the entire column of the torso also act to either stabilize or stress the spine.

Muscle-related pain seems to be the worst in intensity, and the majority of patients arriving by ambulance without major trauma have muscular pain. Muscular back pain is worst in the back, with minimal or no pain radiating to the legs or genitals. Initially muscular low-back pain is usually localized to one side or the other, but with recurrent episodes, the pain often becomes harder to localize. Almost any movement will make muscular back pain worse, and there is usually spasm, which decreases the normal curve of the low back. Despite the severe pain, this is not a dangerous problem, and activity such as walking will usually decrease pain and speed recovery. Without some pain medicine, though, walking is often too painful to consider.

A Battle between Disc and Nerve

A ruptured, or "slipped," disc is one in which the softer inner layer has broken out through the tougher outer layer. If this occurs toward the front of the spine, it may go unnoticed, but if it bulges toward the back, it can compress a nerve root or the spinal cord, causing symptoms.

In disc pain, there is a degree of pain in the back itself, but the more concerning pain and other nerve-mediated sensations, such as numbness and burning, are found in the body parts served by the

26

affected nerves. The commonest pain of this sort is called "sciatica," and the pain of sciatica radiates from the buttock, down the posterior thigh, to the outside of the lower leg. Sciatica is caused by irritation of the sciatic nerve, which is formed by nerves emerging from the lowest lumbar spine and sacrum. The ability to raise the foot and toes toward the shin is powered by the sciatic nerve, and if the nerve is compromised, "foot drop" occurs. Sciatica and other nerve root/disc pain can be persistent, lasting for months or even years at times.

When my father was an orthopedic surgery resident, he would test the patients seated in the hall before back-pain clinic by having them show him the bottoms of their feet. If the patient was able to dorsiflex (pull the foot and toes up toward the shin) without worsened pain, he would let the neurosurgery intern have them because the pain was most likely muscular and no surgery would be needed. If the patient was unable to dorsiflex the foot, or if trying to show him the bottom of the foot caused pain down the leg, my father would have them see the orthopedic intern (his intern—his surgery!).

That was forty years ago, and those symptoms meant surgery. Nowadays those symptoms mean there is nerve irritation, but surgery is not usually considered until time, nonsurgical interventions such as injections, and rehabilitation all fail.

Pain, numbness, hot and cold feelings, and tingling are not considered as serious as loss of strength and function.

When a ruptured disc irritates a nerve root, it becomes a battle. Since the displaced disc material does not belong, it will gradually be remodeled or absorbed. The nerve should win; after all, the nerve is "on its own turf," whereas the displaced disc material is trespassing. Pain and other feelings along the nerve root are caused by the effects of inflammation and pressure on the nerve. If the displaced material causes so much pressure on the nerve that the nerve begins to lose function, the trespassing material may be winning, and an MRI is needed to see if surgery will be required to repair the damage.

The "Battery" of Back Muscles

The human lower back is subjected to more compressive force and more leverage than the spine of a quadruped. Our upright posture also contributes to stiffness and decreased range of routine motion of the back. Sitting, especially with poor posture, is one of the worst things for the back and results in more than one and a half times the pressure on a disc than does standing. In the standing position, a normal spine curvature results in the person's weight being evenly distributed across the disc, whereas sitting causes the discs of the lower back to be "pinched" into a position of greater pressure.

Humans also have a more varied activity level than most animals. Animals in natural circumstances have a consistent activity level. Humans have the tendency to spend the whole week sitting around, losing muscle tone, and then to go out waterskiing after helping a friend move his furniture on Saturday. The decreased tone that results from an inactive week can result in less spine stability during exertion and therefore injury.

The muscles of the low back can be viewed as a battery. Exercises and activity to strengthen the low back charge the battery, and activities to which the back is not accustomed use the battery's energy. Unlike other muscles in the body, when this battery runs out, the back seeks its stability in the form of an acute, very painful muscle spasm.

The low back has the most strength and stability when it is in extension and the least when in flexion (bent forward/rounded). It is important to maintain the standing, extended, position of the low back when lifting and exercising. Low-back exercises and activity increases the strength and tone of the lumbar muscles, charging up the back's "battery" and increasing its stability.

A good example of a very fit back pushed beyond its limit by a combination of exertion in flexion and emotional stress is demonstrated by a tennis pro I treated several years ago. Jake, who was twenty-seven years old and in excellent shape, taught tennis at a local club. One day, he pulled out of his garage to go to work and found that during the night someone had painted graffiti on the lowest section of his folding garage door. He was understandably upset. He decided to see if he could clean it off before going to work. Paint thinner seemed to be working, though barely. He had to squat down while scrubbing hard, shuffling along the door as he went.

As he was finishing, he "felt a sharp stab of pain in the right side of his low back." The pain was the worst pain of his life, and he was unable to stand. He initially fell to the ground when the pain struck. A neighbor saw him lying in the driveway and tried to help him to his feet. He was pale and covered with a cold sweat. Even with the neighbor's help, he was unable to stand. His neighbor called 911.

When I saw Jake, he was in severe pain, lying on his side, and was very vocal in describing his pain as he was moved to the emergency department gurney. With difficulty he showed me the location of the pain—just above the waistband of his white shorts. Palpation of the lumbar muscle was painful. The pain was limited to the lumbar muscle, reproduced with any movement, and it didn't radiate (shoot or move) to the legs or genitals. Jake had no leg weakness, no numbness, and normal reflexes.

I wrote some pain medication down on the order form so Jake's nurse could get it ready, then explained to Jake that the pain, though severe, was not a sign of serious damage and not life threatening. We discussed lumbar muscle spasm and the treatment of a lumbar spasm. I also told Jake that although the shot and pills he would soon receive would help a lot, there would still be pain, and the pain would likely last for at least a week.

The Straw that Breaks the Camel's Back

Most back pain begins with a stress or injury, but it is vital to realize that multiple factors contribute to back pain, and that most back pain comes from a series of stresses, culminating in a "straw that broke the camel's back" phenomena, rather than from an acute single injury.

Luckily the back, and especially the low back, is a very strong structure. Unless there is a defect causing weakness, it takes a lot to cause structural damage to the lumbar spine. Chiropractic manipulations can be performed safely on the low back, and muscle spasm can sometimes be relieved or reduced by this method. The neck, though strong, is not as strong as the low back, and I have seen some serious problems that resulted from chiropractic neck manipulations.

The way back problems are treated has changed greatly over the last ten years, and continues to change. Problems that would have been immediately treated with surgery as recently as five years ago are now often treated with medication and rehabilitation. Good studies have shown that most disc problems respond as well to continued activity and pain medication as they do to surgery. Certainly, avoiding surgery, if possible, is a good idea, since surgery is never without its problems. This success with "conservative therapy" should not be a big surprise to us, since, after all, animals have all along been recovering well from disc problems without surgery, and the structure of the vertebrate spine does not vary much from species to species.

If the pain arose without significant trauma, is muscular with mild or no nerve symptoms, and if you are less than fifty years old, an X-ray will most likely not be done. In patients over fifty with new back pain, spinal X-rays are recommended to ensure there is no unusual problem, such as a bone tumor or fracture.

In the elderly, a seemingly minor fall or injury can cause a fracture wherein height of the vertebral body is lost. An X-ray will show this well, and repair—or at least a more accurate prediction of the duration of pain—will be possible. New treatments of vertebral-compression fracture include "balloon kyphoplasty," in which a balloon is inserted into the vertebral body and inflated, and vertebroplasty, wherein an epoxy-type cement is injected into the bone to solidify and stabilize it. It would be worth asking your doctor about these newer options. We will discuss this again in the "Fractures and Dislocations" chapter.

Addictive medication for pain and spasm, such as opiates (codeine-like drugs) and benzodiazepines (such as Valium), should be used for only a few days at most and then avoided. If such medications are used for a (potentially) longer-term problem such as back pain, addiction and tolerance can become issues.

If back pain becomes recurrent, increased activity, rather than increased rest, is the answer. Both a general increase in activity, such as a walking program and/or swimming program, and specific strengthening and flexibility training for the back and abdominal muscles have been shown to help greatly. Increased exercise will improve the tone of the muscles that support the back and thus will both stabilize the spine and protect it from injury. Increased flexibility will both prevent injury and allow a greater range of movement, while maintaining good posture.

My daughter, a ballerina, can maintain a normal lumbar curvature while touching her forehead to her knee! Increased activity on a daily basis will "charge your back's battery," and add to your endurance as well.

Lastly, there are a few other causes of back pain that your doctor will initially need to rule out. Some of these are serious, and a new, severe back pain, especially in an older person, needs to be thoroughly investigated.

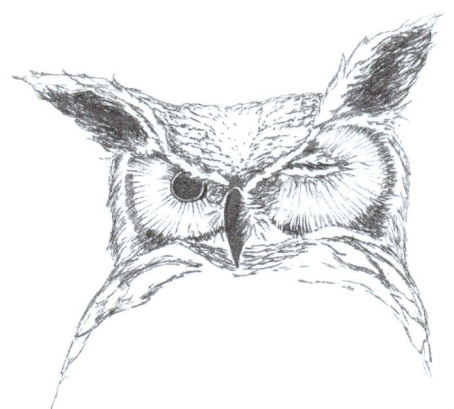

Chapter 5
Bites and Stings

Learn the parts of an insect and you have knowledge. Hold one in your hand if it is wisdom you seek.

—Erin Borden, PhD (Entomologist)

If I didn't have the chance to be a person, I would want to be a fish, or a wave.

—Drake Borden, after playing in the surf, when he was three years old

Bites and stings often are treated in the emergency department. As an emergency physician, I see the initial injury and often infections and toxic/allergic problems that follow the bite/sting.

Medical Wisdom

The statement above, by my son Drake, was made before he was stung by a jellyfish, and "bitten" by a ling cod, into whose gills he had inserted his fingers. His feelings toward sea life have become more complex as he gained experience!

My wife, Erin received her doctorate of Entomology from Washington State University. The kids call her a "bug doctor." Since the commonest bites and stings come from insects, her definition of wisdom fits well here.

Bites and stings can be traumatic, as in the case of a dog or shark attack, or they can be poisonous, infectious, or allergic. Certainly, bigger creatures cause the biggest lacerations and deepest punctures, but luckily (for the victims) they need no venom to be convincing! Smaller creatures, such as snakes and spiders, may cause almost no trauma, but the toxic, allergic, and infectious problems can certainly be serious. Envenomations (when venom enters the body) cause the most dangerous allergic reactions, and even if the venom itself would result in no injury, the victim's allergic response to the venom can be life threatening.

The approach to treating a bite or sting should initially address the injury, then the toxic and allergic effects, and finally the infection and tissue damage.

Serious bites may cause massive bleeding, and this should be controlled with direct pressure. If an artery or large vein is injured, firm focused pressure can definitely stop the bleeding. Applying quantities of absorbent material is an error, and I have seen several deaths caused by this error. Large absorbent pads can hold a lot of blood without stopping or slowing the bleeding at all! Replacing these pads with new ones continues the process of blood loss.

If you stop the blood loss initially, but the bleeding continues when you release the pressure after a few minutes, reapply the pressure. Another person may need to be recruited and taught how to hold pressure correctly while you perform other tasks, such as preparing a pressure dressing, a tourniquet, or calling for help. Sometimes the victim can hold pressure, but if the victim has already lost blood, this is less likely.

A pressure dressing can stop venous bleeding but should be watched closely if used to control the bright, higher-pressure bleeding of an arterial injury. To make a pressure dressing, use an available object or small folded towel that fits the area of the wound and wrap it in place with an elastic dressing. (We will discuss pressure dressings and tourniquets in more detail in the trauma-related chapters.)

To Stitch or Not

Lacerations from bites may need to be sutured, but there is a higher-than-usual risk of infection in these wounds. Any time a wound is sutured, there is an increased risk of serious infection, and this risk must be weighed against the cosmetic benefits of wound repair. In the "Wounds and Wound Repair" chapter, we will return to wound care and cover it in greater detail.

Punctures of all sorts, bites included, should not be sutured (closed), but should be left open. A puncture wound can be defined as a wound that is deeper than it is long. A puncture wound is difficult to clean adequately and should result in minimal scarring anyway.

Cat bites become infected more often than not. An 85 percent infection rate is often quoted for cat bites that break the skin. Not only is the cat's mouth full of tough bacteria, but the needle-like teeth cause deep puncture wounds that are very hard to cleanse adequately.

A good rule to follow is this: "Wounds of less than one centimeter in length should not be sutured." A laceration less than one centimeter long is very prone to be over a centimeter deep and therefore a puncture! Many bites will be punctures. Very small lacerations are not likely to leave a noticeable scar and should be cleansed.

protected, and left to heal naturally. If a small laceration is sutured and contaminant is trapped inside, a serious infection and subsequent scarring will occur. A wound left open will drain (ooze, leak) should an infection occur, but sutures may prevent drainage and force the infection deeper, where it can spread through the tissue layers.

The most common infection I encountered as a medical professor was of scalp lacerations less than one centimeter long that had been sutured. Interns and medical students would feel compelled to place a single suture in such a wound, and sometimes the professor would allow it. Though the scalp when uninjured is thin, the impact that caused the laceration (generally head versus hard ground or coffee table or door frame) causes swelling, which results in a blood collection (called a hematoma) that, when sealed by suturing, results in an infection.

Bite lacerations of the face can be sutured, and the cosmetic result is so important that they usually should be. The greater blood supply of the face makes infection there less likely than on other parts of the body, and certainly scarring there is to be avoided.

Human Bites Most Threatening

Human bites are very prone to infection. The bacteria of the mouth are accustomed to living in the human body at body temperature. These bacteria are also under constant attack by their host and thus must be resistant to the human immune system. Most human bites that occur in assaults don't break the skin, luckily. I have seen many ring-shaped areas of bruising and redness after human bites, but rarely a break in the skin. This is due, I believe, to the bluntness of human teeth and to the fact that healthy human skin is quite rubbery and tough.

Human "bites" sometimes occur accidentally on the athletic field when athletes collide. Occasionally a patient will arrive with a laceration or puncture over the knuckles of the fist, and doctors familiar with trauma will assume that these "fight bites" are the result of a punch to the mouth.

If a tooth enters a joint, a serious infection is likely to occur. Blood does not circulate within the joints, and a bacterial contamination will rapidly become a serious "life and limb" threatening infection. These joint injuries should be washed out promptly and thoroughly. This is often done under sterile conditions in the operating room.

A healthy human can generally bite himself without risk of infection. When I was training medical students and residents, there was a patient who would repeatedly bite himself on the arm, drawing blood, and then call the ambulance. More than ten times he came in by ambulance bleeding, and as human bites are known to have a high risk of infection, he was sometimes treated with prophylactic antibiotics. I had a fun time asking residents if he needed antibiotics, and reassured them that if they had to "lick their wounds" after answering incorrectly, they would experience no additional risk of infection after the self-administered licking! The patient was treated with antibiotics about half of the time, but never got infected.

An individual human's immune system is very thoroughly accustomed to defeating his own oral bacteria. Every time a person chews or brushes/flosses, bacteria from the teeth are released into the blood. These bacteria are immediately recognized and coated by antibodies that are present and continuously created by white blood cells for just that purpose. These antibody-coated bacteria are then devoured by other white blood cells, which are looking for just such a tasty meal. In this way a person's immune system is trained continuously to be ready to neutralize his/her own oral bacteria.

There are times when a human with an impaired immune system becomes susceptible to infection by his/her own oral bacteria, and if these bacteria find themselves in an area with impaired circulation, such as within a joint or adjacent to implanted "hardware" such as replacement joints or heart valves, they can cause trouble. For this reason, prophylactic antibiotics are often recommended for people with implanted prosthetic "parts" when they have dental work.

Licking Your Wounds

Wound licking is instinctual in both animals and humans, and while your doctor is unlikely to recommend it over a good scrub with soap and water, licking or sucking on a wound or cut is much likelier to be beneficial than harmful. Human saliva has been shown to contain at least three antibacterial agents. The tongue is an excellent cleansing brush, and the tongue's sensitivity can allow it to detect very small bits of foreign material, such as a small splinter.

Do not, however, have someone else do the "oral cleansing!" Each person has a different set of bacteria in their mouth, and your immune system is definitely not geared up with the right antibodies to tackle another person's "tough" oral bacteria.

Animals, you will notice, give their wounds an amazingly thorough "tongue lashing." My basset hound spent hours licking the nasty pit bull bite she incurred on her back leg while escaping through a doggie door. She had been stealing cat food from the neighbor's garage successfully for months and then suddenly…a pit bull! I could not suture the wound by the time she came home, since it was too old and contaminated, but the wound healed beautifully, thanks to the thorough cleansing she administered.

Venomous Bites and Stings

Injection of toxin during a bite or sting adds a potential problem for the victim. Sometimes the venom itself is enough to kill the victim, and sometimes the victim's allergic reaction to the venom does the killing.

Chapter 5 Bites and Stings

Most stings and bites do not contain enough venom to kill an average-sized human victim. Why would a rattlesnake, for example, need to kill a human? A rattlesnake is certainly incapable of eating a human. For a snake's bite to save it from a human-sized predator, it would need to be either instantly deadly or so painful that the predator would lose all interest in the snake. Ideally, for the snake, the bitten human would put some distance between it and the snake before stomping, slashing, and striking out in anger.

Bee and wasp stings are one of the commonest, and the injected venom causes burning pain. In the case of bees, the stinger is often left in the wound. This stinger should not be "pinched" but should first be scraped away with a sharp edge, such as a credit card, and then pulled out with tweezers if needed. The venom sac may still be attached to the stinger, and squeezing it during removal will inject more venom.

Most stings will cause some local swelling and redness that occurs in the first hours or day and should not be mistaken for infection—which may occur later. Sometimes this swelling will be extensive and can usually be minimized by prompt treatment with an antihistamine such as Benadryl. Applying ice can also help, and an anti-inflammatory pain medication such as ibuprofen can be used for pain relief.

Elevation of an injured or swollen extremity above heart level is always a good idea. Elevating the extremity will decrease swelling by allowing the blood and fluid to return from the limb more easily. Your body will remind you to elevate the injured part by throbbing painfully when the part is lowered.

Most stings and envenomations do cause a lot of pain, but some are worse than others. Poisonous spider bites have the reputation of being less painful and can go unnoticed initially. Spiders are certainly the creatures most maligned by patients who come to the emergency department. I have seen spiders blamed for just about every problem known to mankind. In reality, an actual spider bite is rare.

In North America our two most worrisome common spiders are the "black widow" and the "brown recluse." Black-widow bites cause muscle spasm and body pain, with very little damage or pain at the site of the bite. On the other hand, the brown recluse causes initial stinging at the site of the bite, followed by blistering, increasing pain, and progressive ulceration (crater-like damage), with tissue loss that continues for a surprisingly long time. Bites of both of these spiders can be deadly, and if you think one has bitten you, try to take it (dead or alive!) with you when you go to the doctor.

Don't Lick that Jellyfish Sting!

Jellyfish sting by injecting venom through a small harpoon-like stinger (called a nematocyst) that cannot be seen with the human eye. Many of the marine stinging creatures are related to jellyfish, and use the same stinging mechanism. If you are stung by a jellyfish, the first thing to do is to remove the "jelly" from the skin. Remove the jelly with the edge of a flat object, such as a credit card. Do not wash the area with fresh water! Fresh water will activate any stingers that are still on the skin, causing them to shoot off their "harpoons," and some will hit you! Instead, wash the area with salt water, or vinegar. Applying heat is a good idea. If it is a hot day at the beach, there may be rocks that can be placed on the wound. Heat can denature (cook) some of the protein in remaining venom, deactivating it. If the jellyfish is one of the more venomous types, such as the Box Jellyfish of the South Pacific, get to a doctor.

A sea anemone has the same stinging mechanism as a jellyfish, but it lives attached to the hard bottom. The stinging mechanism is not as strong, and will not penetrate intact skin of the hands. Sometimes a sea anemone can sting the thinner skin of the forearm, or face, and can definitely sting the tongue! I explained this to a class of SCUBA students, and one student decided to test my advice. He let out a yell and the tip of his tongue became visibly swollen.

Chapter 5 Bites and Stings

Sea Urchin stings can involve venom, but usually are more of a "foreign body" problem. Since the urchin spines are mostly calcium carbonate, applying vinegar (a weak acid) may help to dissolve them. It is hard to get the vinegar in contact with a spine that is below the skin surface, though. When I was diving in Hawaii as a boy I managed to get a dozen or so spines into my right palm. An elderly Hawaiian diver told me to urinate on the spines. This is commonly considered a useful treatment in Hawaii. The acid in the urine may also help to dissolve the spines. There is not much acid in urine, though, and once again it is not likely to contact the impaled spines very well. Removing the spines may be needed if they are in a sensitive area, or if they cause infection.

A sting ray, if stepped upon, can cause a nasty sting. Seen under magnification a sting ray's stinger is barbed, and the venom makes the sting very painful. An injection of a long acting local anesthetic is the best treatment. Heating the area of the sting with hot packs (or hot rocks, at the beach) is especially effective. An x-ray should be taken if there is any suspicion of a broken off stinger in the wound.

Allergic Reactions

Hives are a common allergic reaction that can follow a bite and are caused by histamine release. Histamine is a substance that is released and active in allergic reactions. Histamine dilates blood vessels and makes them more permeable, which leads to swelling. Histamine also causes smooth muscle contraction, which can cause the airways to contract, which results in wheezing and, if severe, difficulty breathing Hives can be rapidly mobile, appearing and disappearing quickly, and generally itch.

An antihistamine (H-1 blocker) such as Benadryl will prevent hives and is even more effective when combined with an H-2 blocker such as Zantac (ranitidine) or Tagamet (cimetidine). The problem is that once hives are present, the antihistamines are not very effective.

This is because antihistamines work by stopping the released histamine from binding to their "receptors." Once histamine release has occurred, it binds very quickly and will not be displaced by the antihistamine. For this reason, antihistamines such as Benadryl and Claritin are best taken before the allergen is encountered. Benadryl causes drowsiness and can be used as a sleep aid. When used for sleep, it will generally work well for a night or two, and then the sedating effect fades. During allergy season, daily use of a nonsedating antihistamine such as Claritin acts as an allergy preventative. Occasionally, hives can become chronic and require extended treatment, but generally they only last a day or two.

Serious allergic reactions are referred to as anaphylactic reactions or anaphylaxis. If hives are accompanied by wheezing, difficulty breathing, facial swelling, or difficulty swallowing, the problem is more serious. "Anaphylactic shock" sounds good on TV and is appropriate, since the reaction causes a loss of the circulatory integrity, a drop in blood pressure, and a loss of tissue perfusion (flow to vital organs). Another dangerous problem is swelling of the tongue and throat, which can impair breathing.

If these symptoms are present, get help quickly. The primary treatment (in addition to the above) is an epinephrine injection. In this situation, epinephrine (adrenaline) is amazingly effective and lifesaving. Epinephrine causes vessel constriction, countering the histamine effect we just discussed. A comprehensive first aid kit should contain both antihistamine, and epinephrine.

Epinephrine is available in a self-injectable preparation called an "Epi-pen," and one of these should be kept available if you (or someone you care for) are allergy prone. For men, the car is a good place to keep the Epi-pen, and for women, the purse is often handy. I have heard many stories where the patient had an Epi-pen "at home" but not available at the time of the sting. Epinephrine will also usually cure even a bad case of hives in about twenty minutes.

Prednisone (a steroid, though definitely *not* the muscle-building type!) will also usually be given if you go to the ER with a significant allergic reaction. Prednisone is more useful in a "delayed hypersensitivity reaction," such as poison oak, than in a histaminic-type allergic reaction, but it may prevent recurrence of an allergic reaction. We will talk more about prednisone when we discuss asthma.

Snakebite Treatment

If you are bitten by a poisonous snake, there is a chance you have received enough venom for the bite to be deadly. This is potentially a different situation than most bites, and the treatment of snake bites has been a subject of a lot of debate. Recommendations have changed over the years.

When it comes to rattlesnakes, the first important point is that when a rattlesnake strikes, and even when it bites, there is often no venom injected. This is called a "dry bite" and occurs up to half the time. Venom from a rattlesnake bite is immediately damaging and thus quite painful. If no pain or very little pain occurs after the bite, it is likely to be a dry bite.

If envenomation occurs, applying a tight tourniquet of the type you would use to stop blood loss is not a good idea, since trapping the venom in an arm or leg could lead to worsened damage of that body part, whereas the body as a whole may be able to handle the insult without permanent damage. No (complete) tourniquet is therefore the best bet in a rattlesnake bite.

When I was a boy I was given a "Snakebite kit" that has a scalpel, and a suction cup. The instructions were to use the scalpel to cut at the bite site, and then the suction cup to remove the venom. I am glad I never had to use the kit. In reality it is difficult to remove the venom with either cutting, or suction, and the cutting is likely to cause additional damage.

Other snakes are potentially deadlier than our rattlesnake. If you are traveling in a country where there are especially deadly snakes, it is worth learning more about them. If the venom is likely to cause death quickly, a tourniquet could allow the patient to receive antivenin and get to an ER before the venom is allowed to reach the bloodstream.

In North America, where it is unlikely that enough venom has been injected to kill the person, the current recommendation is to apply a loose tourniquet, intended to slow the return of the lymphatic fluid (fluid that is outside of the vessels) without completely blocking flow to and from the limb. Antivenin is the key treatment and should be given as soon as possible. Many hospitals do not stock antivenin, and this could cause a delay. Calling or having the ambulance personnel call to confirm that there is antivenin at the destination hospital is a very good idea.

Preventing Infections from Bites

Bites are a major cause of infection. If a tooth, hair, cloth, or other material remains in the wound, it must be removed. Unless the wound doesn't actually break the skin, you can expect your doctor to have the wound scrubbed and irrigated. Proper irrigation involves high pressure flushing. Dribbling or pouring water into the wound is not adequate, and if there is visible contamination, it should be removed by scrubbing. If there is tissue that is too badly damaged to be cleaned and does not bleed when scrubbed, it will need to be removed by the physician. This is known as "debridement."

An X-ray will often be done for a serious bite, and you will not be "out of line" if you ask whether antibiotics are needed. Infection can begin within the first day and seems to come on especially fast with cat bites. Cat bites definitely are more prone to infection than dog bites and need special antibiotics to treat a resistant infection caused by a bacterium called pasteurella.

Chapter 5 Bites and Stings

Infection is a basic problem faced by all creatures, and since it is a damaging and potentially deadly problem we can treat, it is discussed in several sections of this book. Infections of bite wounds are caused by bacteria, and these can come from the biting/stinging animal, or they can be present on the skin and pushed into the wound by the bite.

Infection will not be apparent immediately, and the redness and swelling that occur in the first few hours after a bite or sting are caused either by allergic or chemical reaction or by swelling from the bite trauma. An infection takes some time to develop. Typically, warmth and redness, along with increased swelling and pain, will become increasingly evident after the first day. Oozing of clear or cloudy/purulent fluid will begin and increase. Pus is the remains of dead white blood cells and the bacteria they are fighting.

Once a bite is infected, your doctor will need to decide whether antibiotics alone will be enough to help your body win the battle, or whether additional care will be needed. If there is some foreign material remaining in the wound, such as a tooth, or hair/clothing, antibiotics will not be enough. If the wound was sutured, the sutures will need to be removed and the wound re-anesthetized and cleansed. The wound will need to be "explored," as it will be easier to find and remove the source of the infection than it was initially. The wound cannot be closed again immediately, but should be left open. A "drain" may need to be placed to help ensure that the wound can continue to ooze freely.

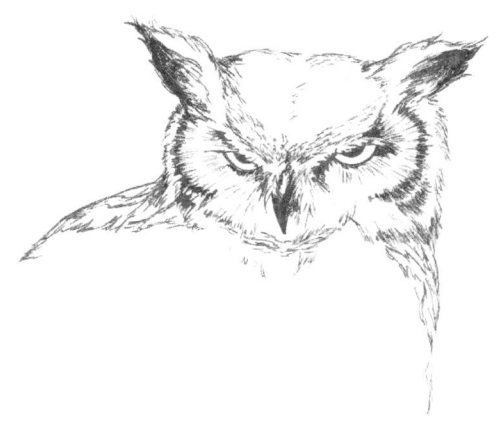

Chapter 6
Bloody Nose (Epistaxis)

"There are a lot of options when it comes to stopping a nosebleed in the ER. Years of experience have shown me that the less I do, the happier the patient…"

The majority of people have a nosebleed at some point in their life. For many people, nosebleeds are frequent and often occur when they have allergies or during dry weather. Nose picking (a.k.a. nostril cleaning/rhinotelexamania) is practiced by almost everyone and often starts a nosebleed. Isn't the word "rhinotelexamania" a beauty?

In more than nine cases out of ten, the fragile network of capillaries and small arteries called "Kesselbach's plexus" is the source of the bleeding. Kesselbach's plexus is located on both sides of the nasal septum. When this is the source of bleeding, it can be stopped by direct pressure.

Medical Wisdom

Applying pressure to a bleeding nose is easy, but a lot of people think they should squeeze the nasal bone. Squeezing the nasal bone will have no effect on the bleeding. Squeezing immediately below the bone is correct, and a firm pressure should stop the bleeding completely. Holding pressure for at least a few minutes will be required, and if you can feel the blood running down the back of your throat, squeeze higher on the nose (still below the bone), and possibly harder.

If squeezing in this manner does not stop the bleeding while you are applying the pressure, you may have a rare "posterior" bleed. If you are unable to stop the bleeding, at least while applying pressure, it is time to seek medical attention.

If the bleeding restarts when you release pressure, you will need to hold it again, possibly for as long as fifteen minutes.

If you come to the ER, the first thing I will do is look to see if the source is Kesselbach's plexus. If the site of bleeding can be seen through the nostril, I will show you how to hold pressure, and you can answer questions with a Donald Duck voice!

I will ask some questions to determine if there is a reason for you to be bleeding. Coumadin (warfarin) is a medication that often increases bleeding, especially when the level is too high. Plavix, a newer "super aspirin" often used in cardiac patients, can also increase the chance of a nosebleed. Aspirin can lengthen the time of bleeding, as well. Even with these drugs, applying pressure is the initial treatment and will usually stop the bleeding.

Your doctor will attempt to determine how much blood has been lost. Typically, blood loss is overestimated, since a little blood can stain a lot of clothing and carpet, but if there has been a long duration of bleeding, or if there are signs of anemia, I will recommend a blood test.

There are a lot of options when it comes to stopping a nosebleed in the ER. Years of experience have shown me that the less I do, the happier the patient. If applying pressure to an anterior nosebleed doesn't stop it after five minutes, I will try ten minutes, and if that doesn't keep it from starting up again when pressure is released, I will try fifteen minutes.

Cauterization (burning of vessels and tissue) with silver nitrate and nasal "packing" are options for stubborn nosebleeds. Before either of these options is used, the nose should be anesthetized and/or decongested with either a pseudoephedrine spray (such as Afrin) or with cotton soaked in local anesthetic.

Cauterization destroys the vessels that feed the nasal septum and will cause septal perforation if performed on both sides of the septum. Cauterization is difficult if the nose is bleeding briskly.

"Packing" has evolved over the last decade, and inflatable balloon-type devices are used more than petroleum gauze. Packing, which is simply another way to apply pressure, will work, but it is uncomfortable. Either a long strip of gauze is "packed" into the nose, or an inflatable balloon is inserted (after lubrication) and then inflated These methods apply pressure to the bleeding vessels from within the nose. Typically the balloon is left inflated for two to three days, but often people cannot stand it for that long. If your nose is packed, you will need both pain medication and antibiotics.

A nosebleed caused by trauma should also stop with the application of pressure. If the nose is crooked, straightening it right away is the best idea. If hours pass and a lot of swelling occurs, it becomes harder to judge straightness, and the nose may need to be rebroken and straightened later by an otolaryngologist (ENT) or plastic surgeon. Sometimes nasal trauma will cause bleeding within the septum, forming a "hematoma" of the septum. A septal hematoma looks like a dark swelling of the nasal septum. If this occurs, the blood clot should be removed to prevent damage to the septum.

If frequent nosebleeds are a problem, they can be prevented during dry weather by applying Vaseline or Neosporin/Bacitracin to the nasal septum with a Q-tip. Increasing the humidity of a house can also help, as can decreasing the incidence of rhinotelexamania!

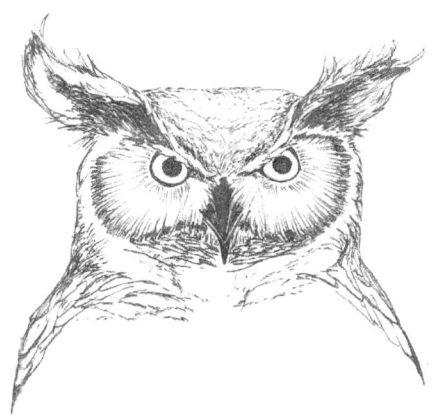

Chapter 7
Burns

There are two types of tissue damage that occur with a burn. The first is the initial injury. Stop the injury as fast as possible with ice or cooling. The second is the nerve mediated inflammatory cascade. Stop that secondary injury, and minimize the scarring with lidocaine (nerve block, and topical lidocaine containing burn cream). The nerve block also stops 100% of the pain... immediately.

—Bo Thomas Brofeldt, professor of emergency medicine, University of California Davis

Few injuries hurt more than a burn. The tissue damage caused by a burn creates an inflammatory cascade, and more tissue damage is the result. It is this inflammation and tissue death that causes the pain.

Pain usually serves some adaptive purpose, and in the case of a burn, the pain is saying, "There is damage happening here! Stop it!"

Immediately cooling the area of the burn with ice or iced water provides instant relief, and burns caused by heat should be cooled immediately. Cooling slows inflammation and reduces swelling. An anti-inflammatory medication such as ibuprofen will provide a lot of relief and should be given early. For severe burns, stronger pain medication will be needed as well.

Burns are classified as first, second, or third degree, according to the depth of damage. First-degree burns are painful and red but do not form blisters. A first-degree burn should leave no scar, but there may be peeling of the epidermis (superficial skin layer).

Second-degree burns involve both the epidermis and some of the dermis (deeper skin layer). A second-degree burn is painful and causes blistering. If the blister is broken, sensitive skin layers are exposed to the air, causing greater pain. If the blister is intact, it forms the ideal dressing and should be left intact. Once the blister breaks, the dead skin that formed the blister should be trimmed back and antibiotic ointment applied. If the blister breaks and is not removed, bacteria can get under the dead skin and cause infection. Second-degree burns take several weeks to heal and may cause some pigment changes, but shouldn't cause lasting scarring.

Third-degree burns involve all of the epidermis and dermis. Third-degree burns may damage deeper tissue as well. Third-degree burns are often dry to the touch, pale or charred, and not painful. There is usually some second-degree burn, as well, though, and these areas are painful. Extensive third-degree burns smell "burned," since the flesh has actually been cooked and is not just injured but dead. Third-degree burns always require medical care. Skin grafting is often required if the area of third degree is more than a square inch or so.

Extensive burns are discussed in terms of percentage of body-surface area, and as the percentage increases, systemic (whole body) effects increase. Even if there is no burning of the mouth, airway, and lungs, if the burn covers more than half the body surface, these areas will swell in the days following the burn, and a breathing tube (artificial airway) and ventilator (breathing machine) will be needed. Most interns and residents initially think it is the inhalation of hot fumes and hot air that causes the airway swelling, but then they realize that after a serious burn, the whole body swells. The body's inflammatory response to a large burn causes increased permeability of vessels, and a lot of IV fluid is needed to maintain blood pressure as fluid leaves the blood stream.

Age of the victim is an important factor in survival after massive burns, and a burn specialist can use the age, as well as the surface percentage burned, to determine when there is no chance of survival. If there is no chance of survival, the large volume fluid replacement can be put on hold, and the patient will be able to speak to his or her family. A large volume of fluid will cause massive swelling of the airway, requiring an endotracheal tube (breathing tube), and people cannot speak when there is a tube between their vocal cords.

Location of a burn is important, and burns that encircle a limb, a finger, or the penis can cause a tourniquet effect and may need a surgical treatment called "escharotomy." Escharotomy consists of long incisions through the third-degree burn to allow tissues to swell without cutting off the circulation.

Second-degree burns to the face, hands, feet, or genitalia should generally be seen by a doctor.

In general, third-degree burns should be seen by a burn surgeon or plastic surgeon; most other burns can be treated well by other physicians.

Burns to the eye present another set of problems, which we will discuss in the "Eye Emergencies" chapter.

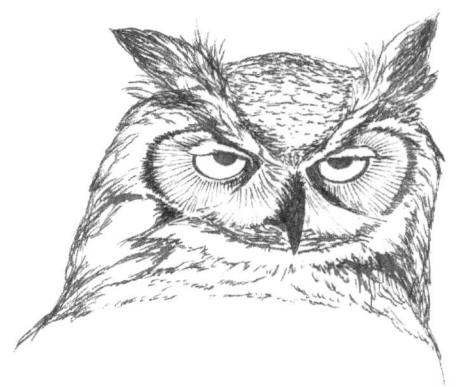

Chapter 8
Cancer

If children have the ability to ignore all odds and percentages, then maybe we can learn from them. When you think about it, what other choice is there but to hope? We have two options, medically and emotionally; give up, or fight like hell.

—Lance Armstrong

Cancer is a general word used to describe when a cell forgets the rules of normal growth and begins to grow out of control. The cell still resembles normal cells in most ways and thus is not identified as a problem by the body. The cells in a cancer are "clones" of the original errant cell and are thus identical.

Tumor and neoplasm are other words used to describe a growth of cells that doesn't belong.

There are many risk factors for cancer, and certainly a main one is increasing age. Since there is no good solution to increasing age, working to eliminate the environmental causes is the best bet in cancer prevention. A tendency toward a particular cancer can be inherited, and environmental factors can cause cancer to arise. Even if all the environmental factors, such as smoking, radiation exposure, chemical exposure, and obesity, are eliminated, there is still a chance of cancer. However, you can shift the odds in your favor.

Once a cancer has started, optimizing your nutrition will not cure it. Remember that the cancer is a part of the body and is identical in almost every way to the body's own cells. Better nutrition will help the cancer prosper just as much as it will help the rest of the body. One of the most tragic cases I have witnessed was the husband of a good friend of my wife's who was diagnosed with throat cancer. He owned a chain of health-food stores and refused medical treatment in favor of holistic and nutritional treatment. As the cancer continued to grow, it became obvious that things were getting much worse, but by the time he sought medical care, it was too late for a surgical cure, and chemotherapy only alleviated his suffering for a few months.

Early detection is important. Colonoscopies and mammograms, as well as the newer blood tests for cancer, are very helpful.

Cancer growths are classified as "benign" and "malignant." Malignant (*mal* means bad) tumors are aggressive and tend to travel to new areas. Movement to another area of the body is known as metastatic spread. Most malignant cancers start small and localized, and if found early, they can often be removed, ending the problem.

We discussed denial previously, but the concept belongs in this chapter as well. It is easy to deny the danger of a cancer and very easy to postpone treatment, but if someone you know is doing this, force yourself to take the time to walk them through a systematic plan of diagnosis and treatment as soon as possible. Nothing could be of higher priority.

The first step is to understand as much as possible about the particular cancer. This step will likely involve sampling (biopsy) of the cancer. A pathologist can tell what type of tissue the tumor is made of and, together with the oncologist, can "stage" the cancer. Staging is basically determining how advanced the cancer is and thus which treatment is most likely to be effective.

Every cancer is different, and some are more amenable to treatment than others. In general, if the cancer cannot be removed surgically, the faster-growing cancers are more easily treated with chemotherapy and other "cell killing" treatments like chemotherapy than are the slower-growing ones. The pathologist will be able to tell how fast the tumor is growing by the number of cells that are in the process of dividing. It is the dividing cells that are killed by the chemotherapy/radiation.

Cancer treatment is advancing, and there are doctors who specialize in different cancers, as well as in different cancer-treatment modalities. I met an oncologist on a plane last year. At the time I was helping to counsel a close friend from my childhood named Scott who had recently been diagnosed with pancreatic cancer. I introduced myself as a fellow physician, and after telling about my friend, asked a few tough questions about pancreatic cancer. The oncologist admitted he was really a prostate cancer specialist and said I should call a pancreatic cancer specialist. Not too many years ago, such sub-specialization didn't exist. Get the correct specialist for your cancer!

Surgery may offer a cure if the cancer is localized and has not spread either into vital structures that cannot be removed/damaged (local extension) or via the bloodstream (metastatic). When a cancer is staged, an effort is made to determine whether it has spread. Sometimes it is easy to tell if a cancer has spread, as other areas are visibly swollen or painful. Sometimes it is not easy, and samples of tissue or lymph nodes will need to be removed by a surgeon and examined by a pathologist to determine whether the cancer has spread.

Surgery for cancer can be either curative or palliative. It is important to understand the difference when surgery is discussed. I frequently talk to patients who return with a recurrence of cancer, and they are often surprised, since they understood that the cancer had been "removed." They believed that the cancer had been cured. When I review the record, it is very clear that the surgery was done with the understanding that a cure was not possible.

My mother required palliative surgery since her bowel tumor had caused obstruction of the bowel. The cancer had already spread to the liver and lymph nodes, so a cure was not possible, but without surgery, life itself would have been unbearable. She did not want major surgery with no chance of cure, and she held off for a little while, but eventually the pain was too much, and the colostomy she dreaded was a blessed relief. In my mother's case, even though the surgery had no chance of saving her life, it was required.

Sometimes major surgery will have little or no benefit, however, and in those cases the surgery itself may be difficult and may not be worthwhile. My friend Scott researched a difficult surgery called a "Whipple procedure" for his pancreatic cancer, and we discussed it in detail. The surgical mortality, even at his relatively young age, was estimated at 10 percent. The Whipple procedure is a long and difficult surgery. Scott decided to have the surgery, and though he is one tough fellow, it was very hard on him. He had a bleeding complication that required another trip to the operating room and blood transfusion. Recovery was difficult, but Scott is still alive a year later and does not regret the decision.

Chemotherapy works by killing cells that are growing and dividing. A cancer grows faster than most of the other tissues in the body and thus is hurt more by the chemotherapy than is the rest of the body. Chemotherapy hurts the parts of the body that are actively growing, such as the hair, blood, stomach, and intestinal lining, in the same way it hurts the cancer. Chemotherapy is often used when removal of a tumor is not possible or when removal is feared to be incomplete. Chemotherapeutic options are constantly expanding, and it is important to have a specialist who is current on the treatments for the specific type of cancer.

Radiation therapy also works by killing cells. Radiation can be used either to locally kill a cancer by killing everything in a certain area or, as with chemotherapy, to kill the more sensitive growing (dividing) cells of the cancer while harming the stable (normal) cells less. "Radiation oncologists" specialize in the use of radiation to fight cancer.

Ideally, cancer treatment will become more able to kill the abnormal cells while sparing the patient. Some newer treatments worth asking about are able to deliver chemotherapy and radiotherapy to the cancer cells specifically. Doctors have long dreamed of a "magic bullet." This seems simple enough, but the problem is that the cancer and the person's own cells are almost identical.

Avoiding cancer is definitely better than treating it. Stopping smoking is such an important step that we should all be jealous of the smokers among us! If nonsmokers could take a cancer-prevention action that is as equally effective as smoking cessation, they could forget about cancer altogether!

Stopping smoking isn't easy, but it is the single most important move that can be made. Not only will smoking cessation reduce the risk of many cancers, but it will reduce or eliminate many of the diseases that keep doctors busy on a daily basis.

There are many cancer-causing agents (carcinogens) to which we are exposed daily. Decreasing the degree of exposure is important.

Sun exposure is an example. The human body is adapted to dealing with, and profiting from, exposure to the sun. The human body requires sun exposure and clearly benefits from some sun exposure, but years of repeated intense exposure will indisputably increase skin-cancer incidence.

It is clear that farmers repeatedly exposed to the chemicals used in pest and weed control have a higher incidence of cancer. It would thus seem that avoiding these chemicals would reduce cancer, but it is not as simple as that. There is likely a "threshold" of exposure that can be tolerated without harm, and as long as that threshold is not exceeded, there will be no problem.

One could assume that the cancer risk from carcinogens is cumulative (as I was taught in med school), and thus lowering pesticide exposure, sun exposure, and smoke exposure would be a good idea. Lowering pesticide exposure might thus allow a greater amount of sun exposure to occur before a skin cancer would result. How to lower pesticide exposure? It might be as easy as buying organic foods or even better, growing your own.

Obesity, or more accurately stated, "having excess nutrients floating around," is definitely a risk for cancer. Cancer, after all, is a new growth of cells, and the gardeners among us will appreciate how much faster a plant can grow when fertilizer is applied. Obesity is in large part genetic, but the overweight person whose weight is stable is in a different metabolic situation than is the overweight person who is continuing to gain weight. If there is a continuing excess of nutrients, there is a risk that these nutrients will be used in an undesirable way. Think about old dogs you have known. Older, overweight dogs have a great tendency toward bulgy lumps and strange growths, while slender dogs don't.

Once the battle with a cancer has started, though, eating enough to survive sometimes becomes the problem. By the time a cancer is discovered, a lot of weight has often been lost. This happens because of a loss of hunger caused by cancer, and weight loss that is not hard-won through dieting is often a sign of cancer. If you know someone who appears pale, tired, and who has lost weight without trying, get them to their doctor fast.

The body is not indestructible, but it is resilient, and it can deal with a lot of damage. The human body deals with many cellular errors daily and eliminates these cellular "slipups" before they become cancers. Optimizing nutrition may not help to cure cancer once it occurs, but optimizing the body's immune system and function can no doubt prevent some cancers from starting.

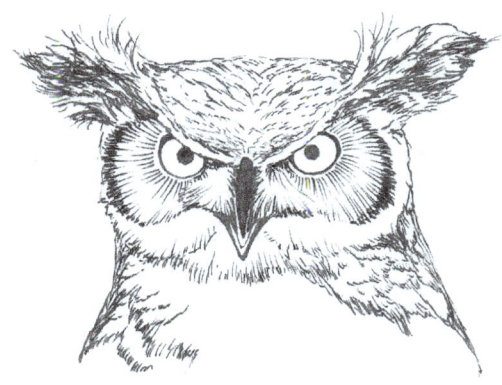

Chapter 9
Chest Pain

The price of freedom is eternal vigilance.

—Thomas Jefferson

Chest pain is, in most years, one of the two leading causes of emergency department visits and generally competes with abdominal pain for number one. Chest pain is a complex problem and has many causes. Most important is determining if the cause is a serious one, which (after making sure you are stable) will be the first goal of the physician who sees you in the ER.

"Chest pain" and "heart attack" are practically synonyms, and the heart is the first thing your doctor will think about. We will first discuss cardiac chest pain and cardiac treatment, and then we will cover other causes of chest pain.

Since chest pain is complex, expect a lot of questions from your nurse and doctor, and be prepared to tell a thorough story. When we talked about abdominal pain, we broke pain down into different types, and the same process is used with diagnosing chest pain.

Cardiac Chest Pain

Cardiac pain that can signal a heart attack, known to medical people as a "myocardial infarction," or MI, is caused by lack of oxygen (ischemia) to the heart muscle. This type of pain is typically a heavy pressure or tightness of the chest. Patients often describe a pressure or weight on their chest that can radiate to the left arm or neck and is often accompanied by shortness of breath or sweatiness.

"Angina" is the same pain, although angina is often used to describe an ischemic (cardiac- caused by lack of oxygen) chest pain that is recurrent and familiar. "Unstable angina" is the same cardiac type of pain, but lasts longer than usual or is more severe than usual. Ischemic cardiac chest pain is likely to occur when there is a greater demand on the heart, such as during exercise or anxiety/stress. Ischemic cardiac pain can often be relieved by sitting down or ceasing activity. Resting lowers the heart's oxygen demand, and if the heart can "catch up," the pain will stop. Age (older is higher risk), smoking, high blood pressure, high cholesterol, diabetes, obesity, and family cardiac history are risk factors for ischemic heart disease.

The heart is supplied with blood by a set of arteries that encircles the heart on its surface. Since these arteries have an encircling, crown-like appearance, they are known as the "coronary arteries." These arteries can accumulate buildups within their walls that cause narrowing. When a gradual narrowing occurs, it can reach a critical point where enough blood can flow to keep the heart working well at a relaxed level, but not enough to supply it during exertion. Exercise-induced (exertional) angina will then occur. Ceasing vigorous activity will usually relieve this sort of pain—though not immediately, since the heart is a difficult organ to rest! If you were loading cinder blocks into a pickup truck, for example, and your right bicep muscle started to ache, you could set down the block, relax the muscle, and the aching would soon stop. It is tougher to rest the heart, however, since it must work ceaselessly.

Sometimes a narrowing that is unstable can then rupture or inflame, causing a clot to form and thus creating a sudden obstruction.

Occasionally a person will be prescribed nitroglycerine, which can dilate vessels, decrease blood pressure, and sometimes relieve anginal pain. Nitroglycerine can lower the blood pressure and cause lightheadedness or passing out, so be prepared to sit or lie down if you take it. Also, good, fresh nitroglycerine causes a headache.

If a person continues to work the heart despite insufficient blood flow, and sometimes just continuing to live is too much work, the heart muscle can be damaged. This would then be called a heart attack, or myocardial infarction (MI).

Sudden Cardiac Death

Unfortunately, a common result of this lack of blood flow to the heart is an "arrhythmia" and sudden cessation of effective heart function, resulting in "sudden cardiac death." If the arrhythmia occurs in the ER, I can generally convert the rhythm to normal, either with medications or with an electric shock (cardioversion). If more than a few minutes pass, though, the heart loses its oxygenation, and the arrhythmia becomes more difficult to convert to normal.

If you witness a "sudden cardiac death," you will need to act quickly. A sudden collapse without warning should be considered cardiac until proven otherwise. Immediate cardiac compressions may stimulate the heart and act to restore a functional cardiac rhythm. A "precordial thump" can be given initially, and though hitting someone is not likely to be an official recommendation of the American Heart Association, it should be. A precordial thump is the best approximation of an electric shock available without electricity.

A precordial thump is a sudden, hard, close-fisted blow to the center of the sternum. Use your hand as if you were doing a karate chop, but with the hand tightly closed. If the first thump doesn't cause the person to noticeably waken/begin to rouse within three seconds, repeat the thump more vigorously. A precordial thump produces ten to fifteen joules of electricity, and within the first half minute or so, this is often enough to restore a heart to its normal rhythm.

If you have had CPR training, you are familiar with chest compressions. The bottom line is to do hard, fast compressions. Realize that what you are doing is pushing down on the sternum hard enough to squeeze the heart between the sternum and the back. The chest needs to sink several inches when you push to achieve that, and compressing the heart takes some muscle. Done correctly, more than a minute or so of CPR is exhausting, and you will need someone to spell you before long.

Atypical Cardiac Pain

Unfortunately, cardiac pain is not always typical. I have seen heart-attack pain of many strange sorts, from a dull ache of the left elbow, to neck pain with shortness of breath. Once such a strange pain is identified as cardiac for a particular person, it may become recurrent in the same atypical fashion and may then be known as an "anginal equivalent." It is safe to say that if you or someone you know has a serious, concerning pain or a strange, new pain associated with shortness of breath or sweating, you should be very concerned and seek medical attention promptly.

Testing in Chest Pain

Cardiac testing is basically aimed at (1) determining if damage to the heart has occurred or is occurring, and (2) determining if there is a risk for further damage. In the following paragraphs, we will discuss the tests you can expect and how they help determine heart damage and risk for further damage.

An EKG (electrocardiogram, also sometimes abbreviated ECG) is usually done shortly after arrival in cases of chest pain thought to be cardiac in origin. Do not be scared because an EKG is done. Your doctor will order an EKG if there is chest pain, even if he or she feels there is only a very small chance that the heart is the cause. An EKG measures the electrical activity of the heart, which provides useful information on blood flow and muscle function/injury. An EKG can in many cases identify a heart attack and can also see stress and lack of oxygen that the heart is experiencing. A normal EKG is reassuring, especially if it is done while chest pain is present.

The EKG has limitations, however, the greatest of which is that it is a "snapshot" of the heart and can change from moment to moment. Continuous cardiac monitoring is generally started, and a change seen on the bedside monitor will prompt the need for another EKG for a closer look. Problems with the heart's rhythm are also studied at this time, and abnormalities in rhythm can be identified and fixed. There are cardiac electrophysiologists (heart electricians) who specialize in problems with heart rhythm.

A chest X-ray is useful in chest pain. A chest X-ray is quick, painless, very low in radiation, and gives a lot of information. It can easily identify lung problems such as pneumonia, lung irritation, or lung injury. A chest X-ray can also evaluate heart size, which can be an indicator of heart disease or heart stress/failure. We will discuss X-rays in much more detail in the "X-Ray and Radiology" chapter.

Blood testing can help to identify if there has been heart damage. Cardiac "markers" are released into the blood when heart cells are damaged. Our newest marker is "troponin." If the heart is damaged by the pain, troponin levels will begin to rise within three hours and will remain elevated for a week or so. Cardiac markers are useful for determining if there has been heart damage, but the absence of a cardiac marker elevation does not mean the pain was not caused by the heart. Heart pain that does not actually cause heart damage will not cause troponin to be elevated.

If the blood, chest X-ray, and EKG are normal, and the heart is not considered to be damaged or in danger, the second testing direction begins. The second type of testing is intended to determine "cardiac risk." The three primary tests in this category are the "stress test" (of which there are several kinds), the echocardiogram, and cardiac catheterization.

The monitored treadmill test is the most basic stress test. The EKG leads are placed (stickers on the chest and limbs with wires attached), and the patient starts walking on the treadmill. A target heart rate is computed, and the speed is increased until the heart is working hard. Since cardiac pain of the ischemic (lack of oxygen/lack of blood flow) type is what we are looking for, the electrical changes that indicate lack of oxygen should appear as the need for oxygen is increased by exercise.

If pain is felt with exercise, the test is stopped and the patient allowed to rest. Pain or the monitor's signs of heart trouble is a positive test. No heart change (other than an increased rate) is considered a negative test. If the test is negative, you will be given a "risk estimate," which may be phrased as "2 percent risk of heart disease during the next ten years," or some such, which is very reassuring.

If a person cannot walk far enough or fast enough to attain the target heart rate, there are chemicals that can get the heart working in a controlled manner. Chemical stress tests can be observed both on the EKG and by an ultrasound (sound wave, seen on a video monitor) evaluation of the heart, known as echocardiography. An echocardiogram can view the heart in motion, study heart-valve function and blood flow through the heart, and see if there is heart damage or changed motion caused by either damage or lack of blood flow.

The "Ultimate" Heart Test

If the above tests should find or hint at problems, definitive testing can be done. Cardiac catheterization, which is done in the "cath lab," is the process of inserting a catheter into the heart and injecting contrast. The contrast dye shows up as bright white on X-rays. A mobile X-ray machine known as a fluoroscope is used by the cardiologist to map and examine the heart and arteries that feed the heart (coronary arteries). Narrowed areas of the vessels can be seen, and action taken to remedy the problem.

This is where the "heart plumber" goes to work. Coronary angioplasty is the process of inserting an inflatable balloon into the narrowed section of the artery and inflating it, stretching the narrowed section, which then remains stretched to greater or lesser extent, allowing blood to flow better. "Stenting" is the process of putting a small piece of pipe into the narrowed area to restore flow and prevent further narrowing. These procedures are trickier than they sound. There is always the worry that small particles and a clot will break off, flowing downstream to block smaller vessels. Small filters are used to prevent this problem.

Stenting and angioplasty are great, but sometimes they are not enough, and cardiac bypass surgery is needed. In cardiac bypass surgery, the blood flow is diverted to bypass the arterial restriction. Sections of nonessential veins are often used to perform the bypass, and these are sometimes "borrowed" from the legs. Bypass surgery is a major undertaking, with frequent complications, and should not be recommended or considered lightly.

Heart plumbing is not as simple as the plumbing in a home. As a nar-rowing of a coronary artery occurs, the body creates new blood flow to the area affected by the narrowing. This "collateral circula-tion" can be enough to maintain the heart. If collateral circulation is adequate, the person should not have pain, and should be function-ing normally. When a cardiac "angiogram" (mapping of the coronary arteries with injected contrast dye) is performed on asymptomatic patients, areas of narrowing are often seen. It is not simple to deter-mine if the narrowed vessels are in need of repair. If there is no pain, and normal heart function, the finding of vessel narrow-ing may be of no importance. Other hints may help, such as an EKG showing (or not showing) stress of the area of the heart served by the nar-rowed vessel. There may be no stress at rest, but a functional test such as a (monitored) treadmill may show important EKG changes.

Upon arrival at the ER, the patient with chest pain will usually be placed on oxygen and often given aspirin. Oxygen can help increase the oxygen level in the blood, and if a part of the heart is low on oxygen from lack of blood flow, at least the blood that is getting to it will supply the most oxygen possible. Aspirin decreases the tendency of platelets to form blood clots. Platelets are small blood compo-nents that in most circumstances are helpful, since they stop bleed-ing. When an artery is damaged, however, platelets can accumulate and form a clot that blocks the blood flow. A heart attack caused by a clot at the site of an arterial plaque (thickening/irregularity) can be helped by aspirin.

If the EKG shows a myocardial infarction (heart attack) in prog-ress, immediate treatment to open the obstructed artery is needed. In hospitals with a cardiologist and catheterization lab, the patient will go straight to coronary angiography, as we discussed above.

Chapter 9 Chest Pain

If the EKG shows signs of decreased blood flow to the heart or injury to the heart, further medications will be given to help increase heart blood flow and decrease the heart's blood demand.

Chest pain can also be caused by a cardiac arrhythmia (bad rhythm), such as atrial fibrillation or another heart irregularity. These changes usually cause shortness of breath, as well, and we will discuss them in the "Shortness of Breath" chapter.

Non Cardiac Causes of Chest Pain

There are many causes of chest pain that do not involve the heart. The esophagus and stomach can cause pain that closely mimics the pain felt during a heart attack. Pain caused by the esophagus and stomach can often be associated with food, and eating can make the pain worse or better. The stomach is able to handle acid well, but the esophagus is not made to withstand stomach acid on a continuous basis, and reflux (heartburn) can damage the esophagus, causing pain. Since the esophagus passes under the sternum, the pain is felt in the chest. Sometimes an antacid can give prompt relief, and while this relief cannot reliably exclude a heart-related cause, it is reassuring.

While heart-related chest pain is often associated with exertion, stomach and esophagus related chest pain often occurs after lying down. A large meal shortly before bedtime, especially if it includes alcohol, is a good esophageal stress test. The pressure of the large meal pushes against the lower esophageal sphincter, and some food and acid will likely leave the bulging stomach and enter the lower esophagus. If pain ensues, sitting up will often bring relief, though the relief will not be immediate. Swallowing some liquid antacid in this case is usually effective within seconds. Another type of chest pressure that increases with lying down is caused by congestive heart failure. We will talk about congestive heart failure in the chapter on shortness of breath.

The lungs can cause chest pain in a number of ways. Lung pain is similar to the abdominal pain we covered earlier. Lung pain can be sharp or dull and easy or hard to localize. If lung pain occurs at the edge of the lung, it will affect the lung lining (pleura). The pleura (thin layer of tissue surrounding the lung) is like the peritoneum in the abdomen. As in the abdomen, pain that affects the pleura is sharp, knifelike, and easily located.

Pneumonia is an infection of the smaller air spaces of the lung. When the pneumonia affects the outer lung surface, it causes sharp pain, increased with breathing. This pain is easy to localize. When it affects the inner lung, the pain is usually less severe, duller in quality, and harder to localize. Pneumonia, being an infection, is usually accompanied by fever, cough, an ill feeling, and shortness of breath.

Pleuritis, or pleurisy, is an inflammation of the lung lining that causes a sharp pain, and though pleurisy can occur without pneumonia, pleuritic pain often accompanies pneumonia.

The chest wall is a rather complex structure, and chest-wall pain can be caused by bone, muscles, nerves, or the joints found there. The muscles of the chest wall can get sore, or spasm, and though this sort of pain is often easily diagnosed by moving or stretching the involved muscle, the pains caused by the muscles between the ribs are harder to sort out. The muscles between the ribs (intercostal muscles) also can affect the nerves that run within them. This nerve stimulation can cause pains that shoot around or across the chest, as well as hot, cold, or electrical feelings—as can the body's other nerves when irritated.

A sharp, burning, or painful area of skin over the chest (or other parts of the body) can be caused by a problem called shingles. Shingles is caused by a reactivation of the chicken-pox virus, varicella zoster. In the case of shingles, though, the virus is localized to a single nerve root (where it comes off the spinal cord), and the infection is limited to the part of the body that particular nerve supplies. The rash of shingles is hard to mistake for anything else, since it is only found on one side of the body, stopping abruptly at the midline. The rash itself usually starts with a few small blisters near the spine, and then spreads outward. In the case of shingles causing chest pain, the blistering rash will continue around from the back, eventually reaching the middle of the sternum, where it will stop. An antiviral medication can help and works best if started early, before the rash becomes extensive.

Last week I treated a seventy-one-year-old gentleman named Peter who developed a burning, constant, and very irritating left-sided chest pain, for which he went to his personal doctor. The doctor did an EKG, a chest X-ray, and blood testing, which were all normal. Peter had been told it was a sore muscle, so he applied Ben Gay. When he came to the ER, his complaint was that the Ben Gay had "burned my skin, and now it is covered with blisters." Peter had the classic rash of shingles, which went from the midline of the back, around to the middle of his sternum, stopping abruptly at that point. When he went to his doctor, the pain of shingles was present, but the rash had not yet erupted. Starting the antiviral early is important, and if a single blister forms with an unusual amount of discomfort, considering shingles is a good idea.

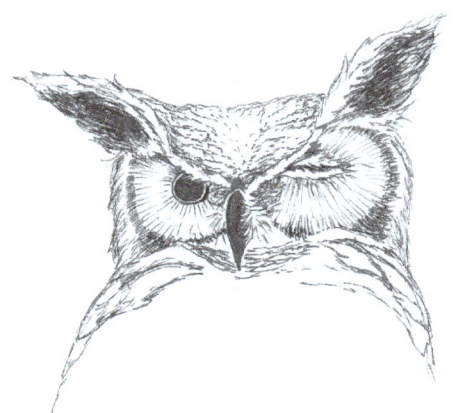

Chapter 10
Cough

"Asthma is well known to cause wheezing, but many doctors forget that a cough is often the primary symptom of asthma..."

Cough is a common complaint and usually means there is a problem with the lungs, trachea, or bronchioles. Most colds are accompanied by a cough, so a cough does not always indicate a serious problem. It is important to know when it is time to worry.

Telling a cold from pneumonia can be tough, as there is some overlap in the symptoms. A cold/flu is caused by a virus, and the viruses that cause a cold/flu infect the entire body. The parts of the body that hurt during a cold are the places where the battle against the virus is localized. A cold almost always causes a syndrome of symptoms, which often includes congestion, sore throat, cough, fever, headache, and body aches. Sometimes a viral infection also causes a characteristic rash.

A bacterial pneumonia, on the other hand, is an infection of the lung air spaces. Pneumonia can follow a virus, and in that case it is called a "super infection." It could be that the secretions of the cold offer a breeding ground for a bacterial infection, or it could be that the immune system is weakened or focused on the cold, allowing the pneumonia to set in.

Generally a cold lasts from ten to fourteen days, and often a cough remains for several additional weeks. Since children in day-care centers catch an average of a cold a month, it often seems like they are "always sick."

Fortunately, after a person catches a cold, he or she develops antibodies that can stop that same virus from developing into an infection in the future. Unfortunately, there are a huge number of different viruses, which means a person can end up catching a bunch of colds.

Catching a cold has sometimes been (erroneously?) associated with exposure to cold weather, and cold season is the winter. Cold weather increases the spreading of a virus by bringing people indoors and therefore closer together. If a dozen people meet in a park for a picnic, and one has a coughing, sneezing cold, it is possible that a few might catch it. If the same group of people were driven into the clubhouse by a cold or rainy day, though, the cold would likely be caught by any person there who breathed enough of the viral particles and whose body was not prepared to combat the particular virus.

The amount of exposure to someone with a pathogen (cause of disease) is important, and even if the exposed person is susceptible to a particular illness, a particular level of exposure is needed to contract it. The mere fact that someone with a bad cough coughs on you does not necessarily mean you will become infected. Assuming you breathe in the viral or bacterial pathogen, most of it will get caught in the mucous of the throat or trachea/bronchioles. The next time you clear your throat, those infectious particles will either be spit out or swallowed. If they are swallowed, they will be burned up by stomach acid and digested harmlessly in the vast majority of cases.

I rely heavily on this principle in my daily work. If I were to catch every disease to which I was exposed, I would be in big trouble, as would my patients. Every day I get coughed on by sick kids and am exposed to all sorts of sore throats and usually several cases of pneumonia. The reason I am not continuously ill is that my level of exposure is generally below the threshold required to become infected. I wash my hands before (and after) seeing each patient, and rarely spend more than fifteen minutes in a room with someone who is ill. Generally, I am wearing gloves when exposed to body fluids and will wear goggles or a face mask when doing dental and other "splash" procedures, such as controlling nosebleeds. By staying below the "exposure threshold" for infection, I avoid being frequently ill and thus avoid spreading infections to my patients.

By now you're probably thinking, "Hey, I already know a lot about that infection stuff!" We keep coming back to the infectious topics because that is a lot of the medical wisdom a healthy person requires.

Coughing up "stuff" is an interesting subject. Many people think that coughing up green or yellow phlegm means an infection, but such is not the case. Phlegm color is mostly determined by how long the material has been around. Mucous starts out white and clear, but then the natural bacteria that live in our bodies colonize it, and the colors develop. Any mucus that hangs around awhile will develop some sort of color. Coughing up bloody or blood-tinged mucous can be a sign of lung injury, cancer, or pneumonia and thus should be taken seriously. Smokers are continually inhaling particles of ash and fiber that must be coughed up, so smokers will have a chronic cough.

How Smoking Damages the Lung

Smoking damages the airway's ability to move mucous up out of the lung and thus causes an increased susceptibility to infection. Smoking also results in very small particles that make it all the way into the deepest air cavities of the lung, called alveoli. In sketches of lung tissue, the alveoli look like bunches of grapes. At this deepest level, the small particles are ingested by cells called macrophages that go around cleaning up material that doesn't belong. When a macrophage eats things it can't dissolve, it basically fills up and dies, releasing its dissolving chemicals into the lung. It is like a war—macrophages against debris, and the lung itself suffers the collateral damage.

The body in this way damages itself by dissolving fragile sections of lung. The walls between the alveoli are dissolved, creating larger air spaces. A healthy lung, if all the surfaces were spread out, would cover an entire tennis court, but the damaged lung has less and less surface area available for gas exchange. As these sections (bubbles, blebs) get larger, the lung loses function, and it gets harder yet to cough out the bad stuff. Emphysema is the result of this process of lung damage. A person with emphysema has lost a lot of lung-surface area and thus cannot get oxygen and sometimes cannot eliminate carbon dioxide (waste product). When we discuss shortness of breath later in the book, we will talk about "air hunger." People with emphysema live a life of continuous air hunger. Looks like a nightmare to me.

If lung cancer were the only risk associated with smoking, I wouldn't waste as much of my time advising patients to quit. The process of lung destruction and resultant suffocation is unavoidable and will occur in greater or lesser degree in everyone that smokes. The only question is whether or not a smoker will live long enough to experience the shortness of breath, and eventual air hunger, of emphysema. Since smoking increases the risk of many other cancers besides lung cancer, as well as markedly increasing heart-disease risk, many smokers die of heart disease before they begin to experience the desperate air hunger of emphysema.

If you are a smoker, please stop.

Asthma is well known to cause wheezing, but many doctors (and asthma sufferers) forget that a cough is often the primary symptom of asthma. If the cough is associated with cold air, exercise, or exposure to an allergen, asthma should be considered as the cause. The most effective rapid treatment of asthma is a bronchodilator such as Albuterol. If the cough is caused by asthma, using an inhaler should give rapid relief. We will discuss asthma and wheezing in more detail in the "Shortness of Breath" chapter.

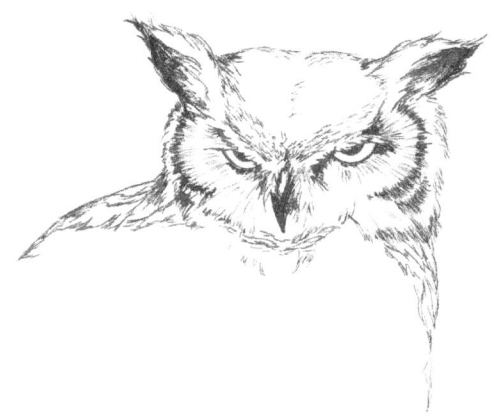

Chapter 11
Death and Dying

The really frightening thing about middle age is the knowledge that you'll grow out of it.

—Doris Day

Life is by nature dangerous. That is the first lesson an education should teach, but education does not teach it, and as a result we have a modern human society insisting on a zero risk environment that cannot be.

—Gene Logsdon, *The Contrary Farmer*

One of my professors would often say, "No one thinks when they wake up in the morning, 'Today I'm going to die in a car accident.'"

Medical Wisdom

I remember hearing that for the first time moments after we declared an eighteen-year-old man dead. He had arrived about fifteen minutes earlier with the paramedics performing CPR. We tried everything in our substantial armamentarium, but could make no progress. What the professor meant was life is uncertain, and we should realize that bad things happen despite our most careful attempts to avoid them. It is easy to deny this fact.

Dead is dead. Though life and death may only be separated by a fraction of a second, the distance between the two is greater than the distance to the farthest star.

The third year of medical school is when students do their first clinical rotations. Before then, I had heard of people dying, of course, but had never actually seen it happen. One of my patients on the pediatric rotation was the cutest little curly haired three-year-old girl I had ever met. Her name was Emily. She slept a lot during our first few weeks together since she was recovering from chemotherapy. Emily had a very unfortunate and completely random (as far as anyone knew) cancer. The punishing treatments she was receiving from us were not helping much, and though we had bought her over a year, she was still going downhill. The decision had been made to offer no further treatment.

When Emily was awake, she was full of life, and since I was a third-year medical student and not good for much else, I had many chances to play with her. She seemed starved for play and would literally wake up, grab some blocks and plastic people, build a structure, and stand them on it within two seconds. She would play and play, enacting all sorts of scenarios. Some of her scenarios involved her family, and many involved her nurses, doctors, and, unfortunately, phlebotomists who drew her blood regularly. She was always short of breath and could only speak in short sentences.

One evening, as she usually did, she took my hand and said, "Got to sleep now," and suddenly flopped down, as she always did. Within five seconds she was asleep, and I could let go of her hand. I taped the pulse oximeter onto her tiny finger, which didn't awaken her. She would pull it off as soon as she woke up, every time. It read 92 percent, which, though low for a normal person, was good for her. I counted her respiratory rate and wrote both on her bedside record. She was breathing a bit fast, but no faster than usual.

I told the nurse at the central nursing station that I was going to the cafeteria and that I'd be back within ten minutes. I knew they were serving tapioca, which was my favorite (and is today, though I gave it a pass for more than a few years after that night). There were only two cups of tapioca pudding left, and they looked a bit old, but were affordable at fifty cents each. I ate them as I walked back to the ward.

When I returned, I stopped at the nursing station, where the ward clerk asked me to confirm an IV rate order on another patient, which I did and signed. Back then I signed my whole first and last name, with MS-3 after it to boot, whereas today it is more of a two letter scrawl. My supervising resident was sleeping in a chair, his feet propped up and fingers intertwined behind his head. More likely he was pretending to sleep. I heard Emily's pulse oximeter alarm start to sound, which usually meant she had pulled it off.

When I got to her, she was lying in the same exact position she had been when I left. The pulse oximeter was still attached, but she was breathing slower than usual, and the reading had dropped to 87 percent. I checked the contact of the oximeter on the finger, which seemed good. Her reading was now 85 percent, and she seemed to be breathing even slower. I shook her gently; no response. Her heart rate was also slowing. My senior resident appeared, and when I began to shake her more vigorously, he placed his hand on my shoulder and said, "It's OK, let her go." He reached over and shut off the oximeter.

Her heart slowed, her breathing stopped, and she was still. Even though a part of me was ready to lose her, I was shocked. I was totally unprepared for the suddenness and finality. I talked about it a bit with my resident, and when her mother and father arrived, we cried together.

Unfortunately, the tapioca was a bit old, and I shortly developed food poisoning, which kept me very busy in and out of the bathroom all night. Eventually I needed an antiemetic (medicine used to prevent or stop vomiting) shot and several liters of saline for rehydration. I am sure the ward clerk and several of the nurses thought I had "freaked out and lost it," but I am certain it was the tapioca.

I had always pictured myself on my deathbed, seriously injured after an MVA (motor vehicle accident), saying, "Tell my wife I love her, thank my mother and father, and tell them that they gave me a great life"...or some such thing. By the time I was an intern, I had seen many critically ill and injured people as they lost consciousness, but had never heard any such noble words. I began to wonder why. Was it that they actually didn't know they were dying? Could it have been that they really didn't have anything to say? Maybe they were too far gone for such noble sentiments. Could it be that their brain function was decreased in the final minutes?

I have thought about it a lot, and I don't think that (at least in such sudden and unpredicted circumstances) people actually really ever believe they are going to die, to end, to just quit being.

While I was an intern on the trauma service, we received two patients from the same intersection. We regularly received serious traffic injuries from that general area, mostly because there are a lot of high-speed roads crossing at right angles and lots of stoplights. Serious injuries do occur on freeways, certainly, but since everyone is moving in the same direction and at about the same speed, accidents often involve many cars with no serious injuries.

In this case, both patients came by helicopter. Both had hit the same telephone pole at about 50 miles per hour. The Life Flight pilot said that when they picked up the second victim, the street was still wet from being hosed down by the fire department after the first accident. Both patients were men in their forties, and both had nearly identical injuries, which included broken ribs, lung damage on the right side, and liver lacerations. Both were talking easily, were oriented, and were able to sign their consent forms to go to the operating room.

I was optimistic as I discussed the surgery with the first man. He asked if there was a chance he would die, and I told him that there was, but that there was also a chance he would do well. There was not enough time for the family to arrive before he was to go to the OR (operating room). I asked him if there was anything he wanted me to tell anyone for him. He said no.

With the assistance of my senior emergency medicine resident, I placed a chest tube on the right side. The chest tube (also called a thoracostomy tube) goes between the lung and rib cage, removing blood and air, allowing the lung to expand once again to fill the chest cavity. Meanwhile, other members of the trauma team were putting in IV lines and a central IV line. The patient was doing better, and no more blood was coming from the chest tube, so we rolled to the operating room.

After the patient was under anesthesia, I held retractors (metal blade-like instruments that hold back the edges of the surgical incision to let the surgeons see), while the attending and trauma fellow examined the liver lacerations and tried to stop the bleeding. We transfused a lot of blood, and fluids were given, but the bleeding could not be controlled and the blood pressure was dropping. Eventually we packed the liver area with gauze to stop the bleeding, and after more blood was transfused and the blood pressure rose, removed the packing (a bunch of gauze pads shoved into the area to apply pressure, and stop the bleeding) and took another look. The bleeding was brisk, and once again the blood pressure dropped and the heart rate rose.

The surgical fellow and surgical attending agreed that the liver damage was too severe to repair and the patient not salvageable. There was so much blood that I couldn't see anything, from my (poor) angle. While the surgical resident closed the incision, the blood pressure bottomed out, the very fast heart rate slowed, respiratory effort ceased, the monitor trace widened from the narrow fast spike of a healthy heart to the wide rolling trace of a dying heart, and the monitor was disconnected. The other intern spoke to the family.

Literally within thirty minutes of returning to the emergency department, we received the second patient. When the reporting Life Flight nurse spoke, it was evident she could hardly believe what had happened. "Same pole as the last patient, front-end damage to the driver's side from high-speed impact, chest injury and abdominal pain are the chief identified injuries." She went on to tell us that the road was still wet from the cleanup from the last call.

Once again, the patient was talking, though mildly short of breath, with some palpably broken (crunchy feeling) ribs and a very tender abdomen. This time it was my turn to put in the central line, which I placed into the right femoral vein, and the other intern did the chest tube. I discussed the upcoming trip to the operating room with the patient, this time advising him that it was a very serious injury that we suspected and he might not survive the surgery. I asked him if there was anything he wanted me to tell anyone. He said, "No, I'll be all right." I wasn't so sure, so I told him that it was sometimes very difficult to fix a liver injury, and that I had recently seen a patient die while undergoing the same surgery. I didn't "pull any punches." I asked him again, and once again, he said no.

The trip to the operating room went exactly as it had with the previous patient. There were severe liver lacerations. Though the bleeding could be controlled with pressure, the injuries could not be repaired. It was my job to speak to his wife and son. They had been told by the social worker that he was in very serious condition, and they had already been crying. I told them the injuries were too severe and there was no way we could stop the bleeding. I would have liked to say more to console them, but could not. I wish I could have said, "His last words were that he loves you both very dearly," but I could not.

Trauma surgical techniques and philosophies have progressed, as we will discuss in the "Trauma" chapter, and those patients might do better today.

I suppose "indomitable human nature" is something we should be proud of, but sometimes it leads to pain. It is hard to distinguish between the invincible optimism we often admire and profitless denial.

Speak to those you love, or write a letter for them to open if anything happens to you. No one wakes up in the morning and thinks, "Today I am going to die in a car crash." Yet every day, many people do just that.

Those deaths occurred almost twenty years ago, and back then the paperwork regarding end-of-life decisions was much less complete and formalized. Nowadays, there is an emphasis on "do not resuscitate" orders and end-of-life forms.

Living Wills and DNR Orders, etc.

A "do not resuscitate," or DNR, order is an agreement between the physicians and patient that delineates the degree of effort and types of actions the doctor will attempt should the patient experience a natural death or serious occurrence that might lead to death if not quickly treated. When I was a medical student twenty years ago, DNR orders were rarely seen and were generally only considered when the patient had an untreatable, terminal disease such as end-stage metastatic cancer. Nowadays DNR orders are often discussed with older patients, even though they do not have an untreatable problem. The reason I say "nowadays" instead of "now" is that I do not want to imply that we have achieved a definitive end point in the end-of-life decision-making process. No doubt the shared thoughts between society and medical practitioners regarding end-of-life issues will continue to evolve.

In mid-2008 my eighty-four-year-old mother-in-law, Charlotte, had a good morning, walking nine holes of golf and managing to drag her hundred-pound German shepherd (who, strangely enough, only wants to stay home!) out for a walk. After getting home, she had lunch and then walked up the driveway to get the mail. Suddenly, she was short of breath and felt her heart racing. Her pulse was fast and irregular. She called my wife, and we advised her to go to the ER. Hu, her husband, drove her there. I spoke to the physician on duty, and she reported that Charlotte had an arrhythmia called "atrial fibrillation," which we will discuss in greater detail in the "Shortness of Breath" chapter. After treatment in the ER to slow her heart rate, she was doing better and was admitted to a large hospital in downtown Seattle.

We visited her that evening. Glancing at her monitor, I could see she was still in atrial fibrillation, though her rate was better. She had not been "cardioverted," had not received the planned anticoagulant they said she needed (instead of cardioversion), and had not been seen by a physician since her admission. She was hungry and still short of breath. She did, however, have a completed DNR form in the front of her chart that specified, "No chest compression, no endotracheal intubation, and NO ELECTRICAL SHOCKS!" Someone had omitted to remember that an electrical shock to restore her normal heart rhythm is what she needed and was why she was there to begin with!

I was enraged, and it was all I could do to remain composed. Swedish is an excellent hospital, probably the best in Seattle, and yet end-of-life paperwork had received a higher priority than patient treatment! She was stable enough that a shock could wait for a bit while the medication had a chance to stop the arrhythmia, but were she to deteriorate... Needless to say, I spoke to the right people very quickly, and nurses and doctors were running in all directions.

In this case, patient care was given a lower priority than end-of-life paperwork. The "pendulum had swung," and swung too far. Charlotte continues to do well today, four years later, and a DNR order still does not belong in her chart. She has no "end-stage" or chronic conditions, is a great and fully competent grandmother, and at eighty-eight years of age can still shoot a better round of golf than I can!

There are times when a DNR order is a valuable document. When a patient who is expected to expire naturally of a known disease or combination of diseases is found in respiratory arrest by the medics (who were possibly called by someone who didn't know better or by a loved one who was gripped by feelings of panic and helplessness) and a DNR form describing a terminal condition is present, extraordinary efforts can be avoided.

When a chronically ill patient is brought to the emergency department, we may have the DNR form available, or the patient's primary doctor may, at times, call ahead to let us know the patient's status. Such patients can be made comfortable, and potentially painful attempts at extending a life that should not, and possibly cannot, be extended, can be avoided.

Life is an unbelievably precious gift. Let's always treat it that way.

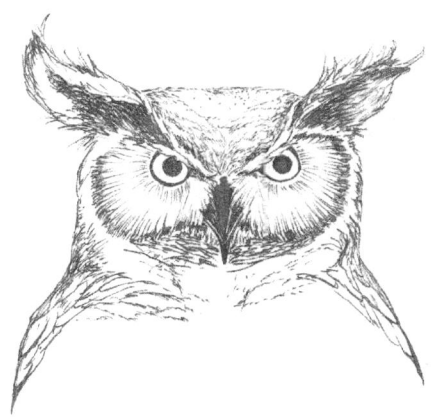

Chapter 12
Dental Pain

*Adam and Eve had many advantages, but the principal one was
that they escaped teething.*

—*Mark Twain*

Dental pain is something most of us are familiar with and does result
in many visits to the ER. Often these visits are in the wee hours of the
morning, when the persistent pain finally becomes too much to take.

The majority of ERs do not offer much in the way of dental procedures. The emergency department can offer pain control and treatment of dental infections, as well as some temporizing measures for
broken teeth.

Most dental pain is not dangerous, but there are exceptions. Decay and infection of the mandibular (lower jaw) molars can become very serious, since these teeth drain into the space below the tongue and floor of the mouth. If the infection spreads to the area beneath the tongue, changing your voice, come in right away. This very serious infection is called "Ludwig's angina" and can progress into the chest and result in death. A fever and voice change known as a "hot-potato voice," which is caused by the tongue being rendered immobile by the infection beneath it, is typical of Ludwig's and requires immediate antibiotics and surgery.

If a tooth is completely knocked out, it should be promptly replaced in its socket. By the time you come to see me in the ER, it will be too late for the tooth to survive. Ideally the tooth should be replaced within five minutes, and if it is replaced immediately, it will be easier to seat it well within the socket. If the tooth is dirty, gently cleanse it before replacing. At that point, you will need to go to the dentist or to an oral surgeon to have the tooth stabilized in place while it heals.

A fractured (broken) jaw is painful, often requires surgery, and makes it very difficult, if not impossible, to chew something solid. A test I use to see if the mandible is broken is called the "bite test." I have the patient bite down on a tongue depressor, first on the right side, then center, and finally left. If the patient can bite down hard enough to break, or stop me from removing, the depressor, it is unlikely the jaw is broken. From this you can infer that if you can chew well, the likelihood that your jaw is broken is very low.

When it comes to dental pain of the type caused by decay, whether it is the initial damage to the weakened tooth or pain from a lost filling, there are a number of options.

If the painful root/area is exposed, a number of things can be applied to the tooth. One that is especially effective is a cough medicine called "tessalon perles." These liquid-filled capsules can be punctured, and the contents squeezed out on the painful tooth. Ambesol can also work in this fashion.

Pain medication such as aspirin or ibuprofen can help somewhat, and for a short period, stronger pain medication such as codeine or hydrocodone can be used. Since tooth pain is often recurrent and can be persistent until treated, narcotics and other addictive medications should be used on a very short-term basis for dental pain, if at all.

A dental nerve block can be done by many or most emergency physicians and is by far the best way to get complete pain control. A nerve block with the longest-lasting local anesthetic can give complete pain relief for six to eight hours, and usually, by the time the nerve block begins to wear off, the worst pain is over. Long-lasting nerve blocks are also proven to have a lingering effect that can reduce pain for days or weeks after the injection.

A dental abscess may need to be drained (opened, lanced). A dental abscess causes swelling of a particular area, and sometimes there will be a foul smell or pus. Normally a nerve block or local injection will be done first, and then an incision or aspiration is performed to give the infection a route of exit.

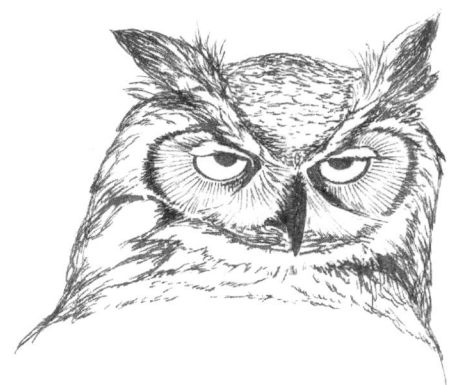

Chapter 13
Diet and Exercise

One can never be too fit, or have too much compost.

—James Borden, MD

Many books have been written on diet and exercise. If you listen to the radio or watch TV for even a brief time, you will see weight-loss ads with all sorts of wild ideas and interesting promises. Clearly, losing weight and getting toned is a popular goal, and many people think about losing weight every day. Inadequate nutrition is not as big a problem in the developed world these days as is "over nutrition."

In this chapter I will not advocate any particular diet program, but will instead tell you the basic facts about nutrition and weight loss. I will mention some nutritional aspects of a few diet plans, but mostly you will be able to decide, after reading this chapter, if a particular plan is medically sound and likely to work. Some diet plans, such as Atkins (dropping carbohydrates), definitely result in weight loss, but are not sustainable for most people, and the weight returns.

There are essential nutrients and vitamins/minerals that everyone needs. Protein is essential, as are some fats. Many vitamins are needed. It is impossible for a human to be a pure vegetarian without supplements and still retain good health. With vitamin supplementation, including B-12, it is possible to eat only plant products and remain healthy.

There is much debate regarding how much protein is needed per day. Generally the consensus is one to two grams per kilogram of body weight. Protein is "essential" because the body is unable to manufacture nine of the twenty required amino acids (there are nine essential amino acids). The amino acids (building blocks of protein) are found in variable amounts in different foods, and combining foods properly makes a more efficient diet. Beans and rice are two foods that complement each other nicely. Rice, and other grains, are poor in the amino acid Lysine whereas beans, peas, and legumes are rich in Lysine. When I first began raising poultry for food I was worried that the birds would not grow well on our homegrown grain. I have not mastered growing enough tons of any legume to feed the birds yet, but I have plenty of barley and wheat. It was with trepidation that I fed the turkeys only barley during that first year, but they did fine. They were able to eat grass every day, and a few insects/worms as well, which helped. They grew slower than if I had added a legume to their feed to balance the amino acids, but they reached full size and their superior flavor resulted in a high demand. I am certain that in their "search" for Lysine they consumed more pounds of grain (more calories = more waste) than they would have with supplementation. Meat (animal protein) contains a balanced full spectrum of amino acids and other nutrients so my birds of prey (owls included!) require little if any supplement.

Carbohydrates are not essential, as Atkins dieters learn. Good carbohydrates do supply quick energy, can supply roughage, and are tasty to eat. There is a lot of variability in carbohydrates, and while some of the bleached, processed grains have little but energy to offer, a high-quality, pesticide- and herbicide-free whole grain has substantial nutritional benefit and is more satisfying. Fruit Juice that has been filtered, pasteurized and stored in bottles or cans offers little but energy content, and cannot compare with fresh, whole fruit.

Taking at least some vitamin supplement is not a bad idea. If you don't need the vitamins, they will be quickly eliminated and go down the drain. This is easy to demonstrate if you do not already take vitamin pills and have a borderline diet. Just go buy a good-quality adult multivitamin and mineral supplement. Take one in the morning and watch your urine. Chances are it won't change noticeably in color. Continue to take one each day, and continue to watch your urine. When your body has loaded up on B-2, also known as riboflavin, the excess will be dumped. Your urine will turn noticeably bright yellow. The yellow is a different yellow than usual and almost looks fluorescent. You can then decrease the vitamins to every other or every third day. Possibly, if you are eating well, only one a week will be needed.

This is not a scientific way to ensure perfect vitamin intake, because we are relying on a single "marker" vitamin. If the supplement is balanced, though, it should come close. There is no downside to taking one each day as directed, other than added expense and waste. If you are low on B-vitamins you will feel more energetic within the first day. If you were fine before adding the supplement, you will notice no difference.

Medical Wisdom

As you can gather from the above, the body has an ability to retain more of a given nutrient and can increase its ability to hold onto a nutrient that is in short supply. "Total iron-binding capacity" is a test that evaluates how much iron the blood can potentially bind. When there is plenty of iron, the binding capacity is decreased, and iron is allowed to escape. When there is less iron available, the binding capacity is higher, and iron is grabbed up when available. The body must be given a chance to get the nutrient it needs. If there is inadequate iron intake, even a high binding capacity will not result in adequate stores.

While sun exposure is known to increase the chance of skin cancer, the risk of not getting enough sun is also serious. Without adequate vitamin D and calcium intake and some sun exposure to convert the vitamin D to its active form, bone weakness and, in children, rickets (bent and weak bones) can result. There have actually been more cases of rickets in developed countries with the avoidance of sun exposure and increased use of sun block. If you are a sun lover, the next time someone accuses you of "trying to get skin cancer," you can counter with, "and are you trying to get a broken hip?"

Weight control is a major business in the world today. If losing weight and remaining slender were easy, weight loss would not be a multibillion-dollar industry.

Body weight is largely determined genetically. Some people eat whenever they feel like eating, as much as they feel like eating, and yet do not become obese. Others in the same "give no thought to diet" situation will become very obese. Fighting this genetic tendency to be a certain weight is possible, but not easy. Changes in food intake and activity level can make anyone lose or gain weight. Realize, though, that when you step on the "dieting treadmill," you will not be able to step off without gaining back the lost weight. Maintaining a weight below your body's natural genetic "set point," once you have lost the weight, will require continued dietary restriction and/or lifestyle change.

Chapter 13 Diet and Exercise

Food Energy – Calories

The energy in food is rated in kilocalories, usually referred to as "Calories." A Calorie is an actual amount of energy. One Calorie is enough energy to raise the temperature of one liter of water by one degree Celsius. The human body is a machine that requires energy to run, and this energy comes from food. Burning food (drying it out and actually lighting it on fire) will release the energy as well.

If you wanted to do an experiment, you could dry out a piece of toast and use it as a small piece of "firewood" to heat up a pot of water. If you put one liter of water in the pot and carefully measure the water's temperature increase after the "toast log" is burned, you could calculate how many calories the toast contained. If the water went from a cold 10 degrees Celsius to hot 110 degrees Celsius, the piece of toast would contain 100 calories. The scientists among you are saying, "Remember, some heat goes into the metal of the pot, and some is lost into the air." True, but if we could measure all of that heat and apply it to the water, we would have an accurate measure of the Calories in the toast. Calories are actually measured this way, by burning the food item in a "combustion chamber" and measuring the heat output.

Gasoline has a certain amount of stored energy that is released when it is exploded within a car's engine. Some of this energy is used to move the car forward. The human body works in the same way—"exploding" the chemical bonds in food to produce the energy it needs to stay warm and move forward.

The average 125-pound woman needs about 2,000 calories a day to maintain her weight. The average 165-pound man needs about 3,000 calories a day to stay at an even weight. From these numbers, an inactive person should subtract about 500 calories a day and an active person add accordingly. One pound of stored body fat contains 3,500 calories.

An excellent article on the facts of fat was written by Dr. Doug McGuff, MD, titled "Body Fat: Hard Facts About Soft Tissue." It is easy to find online.

The Mechanics of Weight Loss

Weight loss is every bit as simple as putting gas in a car. If your car holds twenty gallons of gas and gets twenty miles per gallon, you can drive it four hundred miles on a tank of fuel. Since gas weighs about seven pounds per gallon, if you drive your car a hundred miles, it will burn five gallons and lose about thirty-five pounds. If your tank only has five gallons in it, and you fill it up to twenty, your car will have gained one hundred and five pounds at the pump. If a person burns more energy than he or she takes in, and does it consistently, he or she will lose weight.

Increased activity results in increased calorie burning, and more food needs to be eaten to maintain the same weight. You don't need to say at dinner, "Let's see, I ran an hour today, which burns five hundred calories, and therefore I need to eat two extra scoops of rice." Your body knows you need to eat more and will automatically do so unless you consciously stop eating and remain hungry. If you don't make up the burned five hundred calories at dinner, you will be extra hungry at breakfast the next day; if you don't get the food at breakfast, you will have a strong tendency to eat a bigger lunch; and so on.

Exercise is indisputably healthy. People feel good after vigorous exercise. Weight training and aerobic (breathing hard) exercise combined is the best. Increasing the muscle poundage increases the body's daily caloric need, whether or not the muscle is being used, because muscle is more active and uses more energy than fat does. Active, toned muscle also burns more energy than soft muscle. Exercise definitely stimulates the appetite. If exercise didn't naturally stimulate the appetite, life-threatening weight loss would soon sideline all serious athletes, especially endurance athletes! How much exercise is ideal for health and longevity is a long-running debate, pun intended! But it is clear that exercise is beneficial in many ways.

Most people, if asked why obesity is becoming a "big problem" in society (once again pun intended), will reply, "People don't need to work as hard physically these days; they have machines to do their work." That is not the real problem, however. The real problem is the abundant, refined, calorie-dense food everywhere we look. If a hungry person had to get their calories from apples and lettuce (bulky, fiber rich, unrefined), rather than from hamburgers, cookies, and muffins (refined, oily, dense), it would be a lot harder to gain weight. One large hamburger, for example, can equal ten apples in calorie content. I don't know about you, but I can eat two of those hamburgers easily. Have you ever tried eating twenty apples? One hamburger might cause constipation, but let me tell you, eat ten apples, and constipation will be a long-forgotten problem! Fiber is what makes the difference.

Working hard on the farm all day, from dawn to dusk during harvest, I might burn an extra eight hundred calories! I can eat eight hundred extra calories at dinner in only a few minutes, and I do because I am very hungry. I am also very thirsty and can drink the eight hundred calories by having a few cups of "fresh-squeezed" chocolate goat milk in seconds. Squeezing the milk out of the goat also burns calories, but my wife, Erin, usually does the milking.

Why Fat?

The human body is amazingly good at maintaining itself in a steady state. Fat storage has ensured the survival of human beings during hard times, drought, famine, disease, and cold winters through the ages. Through all but very recent human history, starvation was the threat, and obesity was a form of wealth. Having some fat stored is like having a cupboard full of canned food. The only problem is that with fat, you can't leave the cans at home when you go to the beach! Starvation is still a bigger problem than obesity in parts of the world, and in those places is a far deadlier problem than obesity will ever be, anywhere.

The bottom line, if you want to lose weight, you will need to feel some hunger. It also has to be a sustained effort, going from day to day and year to year. It takes a real commitment.

Satiety and Fasting

Some foods satisfy hunger better than others, and those can be used as snacks. A handful of nuts, which is about a hundred calories, for example, will satisfy hunger a lot better than one cup of apple juice or six pieces of candy, which may also be a hundred calories.

Fasting is an interesting process and helps with an understanding of the body's workings. Many people eat multiple meals every day and begin to think that if they miss a meal, something serious may happen. I often hear, "I was so hungry, I thought I might pass out." There is nothing wrong with an adult missing some meals. As a matter of fact, it is probably very healthy to miss meals. A leading cause of adult-onset diabetes is the continuous abundance of calories entering the bloodstream. Insulin is constantly the dominant hormone as it works to "pack away" the excess nutrients.

If you were to skip food for three days (assuming you are in normal health) here is what would happen. (You will continue to drink water—and enough water to stay well hydrated—but no other types of liquid.) You would feel hungry before too long, and food would look good. If you looked at it and thought about giving up on the idea of fasting, your stomach would feel even hungrier and might growl a bit. That sound is your stomach preparing to receive some food! If you had made the firm decision, though, that you were not going to eat, period, the hunger would be less. By the end of the first day, the hunger would be decreased. By the second day, you would feel much less hungry. Food would still look good, but knowing there is no chance of eating any would decrease your hunger.

Most people start to feel really good on the second and third days. You would have more energy, feel lighter on your feet, and your vision would seem sharper. Your hands might feel a bit colder, as your body tried to conserve heat (conserve energy/save calories) by decreasing the blood flow to the arms and legs, where the most heat is lost. The body would tighten up the ship, conserving energy in any way possible, and fat burning would become a primary process. Burning fat releases ketones, which would cause a change in the smell of your breath. A man who normally burns 3,000 calories a day can, by becoming metabolically more efficient, decrease to a requirement of less than 2,000 per day. At the new 2,000 calories-a-day requirement, you would still be losing more than a half pound of fat a day, though. When it came time to break the fast, you would be surprised to find that you were not actually very hungry and could easily continue to give food a "pass."

There is no harm in such a fast. There is usually no permanent weight loss either, because once you start eating, you will find you are much hungrier than usual, and you will, if not careful, quickly make up for the missed calories.

The Empty Calorie Concept

"Empty calories" is a concept worth remembering when we talk about diet and nutrition. Soft drinks contain a lot of sugar (carbohydrate) calories, but they contain no protein, fat, or vitamins. A huge-sized sugary soft drink may contain eight hundred calories, but a much better nutritional choice would be two apples, a banana, a can of tuna, some broccoli, some carrots, and a big glass of water—for the same eight hundred calories. Eating a lot of empty calories will not replace the good food your body needs. The craving for essential nutrients will still be there, and the eight hundred calories will just add to it, practically guaranteeing a daily caloric excess and weight gain. If a teenage girl, for example, drinks four cans of pop a day and gets the other thousand calories from food containing nutrition, those other thousand calories had better be nutritionally rich and balanced, because they need to supply the day's nutritional needs. Elimination of empty calories will help weight loss, and health in general.

For a person with the genetic tendency, it is actually very easy to become obese. Say a 130-pound woman eats an extra piece of toast every day for breakfast, while also consuming her usual weight-maintaining diet. A small piece of toast contains about 100 calories. That means she will eat an extra 3,000 calories in a thirty-day month. Since a pound of fat contains 3,500 calories, she will gain 10 pounds a year (lost a few crumbs!). During high school and college, she would gain 80 pounds of fat and weigh 210 pounds! One extra piece of toast a day does not make her a "glutton"; no one would watch her and say things like, "Wow, watch her pack it away!"

It is equally hard for a person with the genetic tendency to be slender to gain excess weight. In studies involving young, slender people who were forced to eat extra food every day, which was carefully recorded, they did gain weight as expected. They did not feel like eating the extra food, but did so out of obedience to the program. When the study was over, they did not try to lose the weight, but the weight came right off naturally, and they returned to their pre-experiment weight.

Diet and Life Extension

Longevity and life extension is important to all of us, but extension of the active and productive life span is the key, rather than just adding years. There has been only one scientifically proven way to extend the active, healthy life span of mammals, and that is caloric restriction. If two groups of animals of the same age and species are isolated, and one group is given all they want to eat, while the other is given only a bit more than half of that eaten by the first group, the caloric-restricted group can live almost twice as long! Possibly of more importance is the higher activity level and better health in general of the calorie restricted group.

I learned about this diet in my first year of medical school at Case Western Reserve University. The professor told our class that "caloric restriction is the only proven method of extending active lifespan." I read as much as I could find, was convinced, and then decided to give it a try.

I carefully tracked my caloric intake for a week, and, taking 60 percent of that amount as my restriction goal, came up with 1,800 calories per day. This level of restriction was no small change in lifestyle. I ate very healthy food, ensuring that I got at least 100 grams of protein per day, as well as adequate fruits and vegetables. I also took a daily vitamin pill.

Since I was in med school, this was an easier time to follow such a diet. Erin and I were short on money, short on time, and didn't have kids to feed (and therefore eat with). Erin was working as a college professor at the time and training for the Hawaii Ironman Triathlon, which she qualified for—and finished—twice.

I started the diet at 164 pounds and five feet nine inches. After the first week, I noticed that my hands and feet were cold all the time. My weight had dropped by several pounds, and I felt very good. By the end of six months, my weight had stabilized at a muscular 152 pounds, with very little fat. I still felt very good. I felt better than I ever had before, as a matter of fact, but I wore warmer clothes.

Eventually I "fell off the wagon." I don't remember how it happened, but it probably had to do with the long nights in the hospital, with all of those snacking temptations and stress. My weight rose back to the low 160s over the following year. Twenty years later, my weight is 164 pounds again on an average morning. I do intend to restart the diet on my fiftieth birthday, which is now less than a year away. I do recall that it was hard to eat less, but I also remember how delicious the food tasted.

Obesity is definitely damaging to the body structure. Knee replacements are difficult for the orthopedist and difficult for the patient, but are needed much sooner in the obese patient. Obesity contributes to cancer (as we discussed in the cancer chapter), heart disease, diabetes, and a host of other problems. As an emergency physician, I do not know enough about the newer stapling and banding (bariatric) surgeries to give advice on them. I see a fair number of complications from those surgeries in the ED, though, so I know they do have some risks. If you are dangerously obese, it is probably worth knowing all the options and going in for a consultation.

A combination of ensuring adequate exercise and decreasing caloric intake over a period is a key to healthy weight loss. It is hard to eat while jogging, just as it is hard for me to spend "my wife's money" on farm supplies while working in the ER! Realize that, as Winnie the Pooh says, "A bear, no matter how hard he tries, grows tubby without exercise." Also realize, though, that as Winnie the Pooh later says, "Up, down, up and down puts me in the mood…for food," and prepare to resist that natural appetite stimulation.

It is proven that keeping a graph of your weight and weighing yourself daily helps. Possibly, this acts as a daily reminder and encourages a renewal of commitment. Dividing the day into sections also helps, since it is easier to stick to a resolution for three hours, than it is for six!

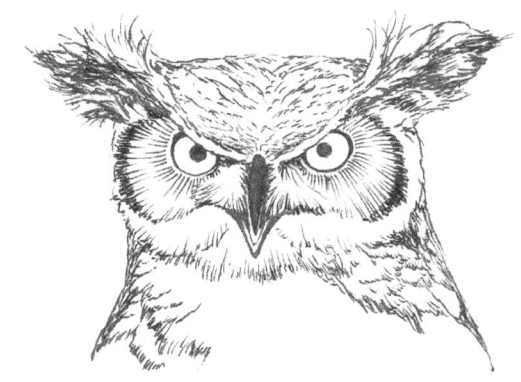

Chapter 14
Dizziness and Vertigo

*For a man to attain to an eminent degree in learning costs him time,
watching, hunger, nakedness, dizziness in the head, weakness in the
stomach, and other inconveniences.*

—**Miguel de Cervantes Saavedra,** *El Quijote,* **circa 1600**

The first series of questions your doctor is likely to ask when you complain of dizziness is aimed at distinguishing between the "light-headed" sort of dizziness and the "I am spinning" or "the room is spinning" sort of dizziness. The first type can be caused by a number of things, and the second is called vertigo.

Vertigo

Vertigo can be of a number of different types, and it can be severe and debilitating. The most severely symptomatic vertigo is, strangely enough, also the least indicative of a serious problem. When a person has a sudden attack of vertigo, it seems as if the room is spinning out of control. Walking is nearly impossible, even when holding onto a wall, and vomiting or severe nausea often occurs.

Benign positional vertigo is the commonest type and comes on suddenly with a change in head position. "Benign" refers to the long term, since it certainly isn't benign in the short term! In the inner ear are a series of tubular structures called "semicircular canals." These structures are partially fluid filled and have small sensors to detect the position of the fluid, which then tells the brain which way gravity is pulling and therefore which way is down. Presumably, the fluid can thicken at times, or small particles can detach and move around, and some can remain adherent to the sensors in another part of the tube, sending "down is up, up is down!" messages to the brain. This sort of sudden-onset, severe vertigo is rather common, and since it is so severe, many people come to the ER the first time they experience it.

Sometimes maneuvers can relieve this sort of vertigo. There are a variety of vertigo maneuvers, but they are all intended to move or shake the semicircular canals, freeing up the sticky liquid or particles so that gravity and movement can once again be interpreted correctly. The maneuvers I usually use involve having the patient sit on the edge of the bed and fall onto pillows first to the right side so that the right ear hits the pillow first, then onto the left side so that the left ear hits first. Next the face hits to the left, then to the right, and finally the patient falls backward so that the back of the head hits the pillow. Usually a practice run is needed for each fall so that the second one has enough speed and impact. These maneuvers can cause vertigo in a person who is prone to it, or cure it in a person who is suffering from an acute attack.

Medication options for vertigo also exist. Meclizine, also appropriately called Antivert, is often effective and usually reduces the severity at least. If meclizine fails, one of the benzodiazepines such as Ativan or Valium will often be successful. Sometimes both will be needed.

A more gradual onset of generally milder vertigo can be much more serious and can indicate a more difficult problem, such as a cerebellar (posterior brain) tumor. Vertigo combined with ringing in the ears and hearing loss indicate possible Meniere's disease (an inner-ear disorder). See your doctor if you have gradual or progressive symptoms, or if the problem fails to go away completely.

Lightheadedness

The other sort of dizziness is often described as lightheadedness or "feeling like I might pass out." Actually passing out is important to report, and we will discuss that in the "Syncope and Seizure" chapter. Lightheadedness generally indicates there is less blood getting to the brain than normal. Sometimes lights will flash before the eyes when this blood flow drops, since the eyeballs are under a degree of pressure and thus the blood needs to have a higher pressure to get into them. Dehydration is a common cause of this sort of dizziness, and a faster-than-usual resting pulse may be a clue.

The heart itself can cause decreased flow and resultant dizziness when weakened or inefficient for some reason. An arrhythmia causing it to beat too fast or slow, a valve problem, or a small heart attack are a few examples of things that can weaken the heart. If you are dizzy and think it may be your heart, call or get to your doctor or the ER right away. If your pulse is less than sixty or more than one hundred beats per minute, and dehydration is not to blame, think the heart.

Sometimes a new blood pressure medicine can "overshoot," lowering the blood pressure to the point where someone feels dizzy.

Medical Wisdom

If this occurs, the dizziness often comes shortly after the medication is taken and may be most pronounced when the person arises from a seated or lying position to a standing position. If this occurs, a smaller dose may be needed. I see a lot of people with head injuries and even broken bones from falling when they feel lightheaded, and many physicians, including myself, think that leaving the blood pressure a wee bit on the higher side of normal is a safer plan.

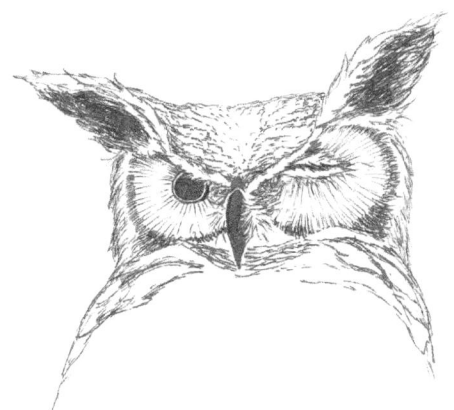

Chapter 15
Drowning and Near Drowning

*One never dives into the water to save a drowning man more eagerly
than when there are others present who dare not take the risk.*

—*Friedrich Nietzsche*

Many misconceptions about drowning exist. One misconception is
that drowning is a loud event, heralded by much hollering and splashing. In general, nothing is further from the truth. Drowning is usually
silent and can go completely unnoticed, even in a crowded pool.

A tragic example of this occurred at the Davis Athletic Club in
Davis, California, in the summer of 2000. Even though there were dozens of adults and scores of children playing in the pool, an eight-year-old

managed to slip silently beneath the surface within a few feet of the water's edge and drown. Even though one of my university colleagues, a fellow emergency physician, was present, the child's disappearance went unnoticed just a few minutes too long, and she could not be resuscitated. This was a horrible tragedy, which deeply affected many people.

Another misconception is that "lots of water is breathed in, and the most important thing is to get that water out." This is untrue. Usually no water, or a very small amount at most, is breathed in, and then the airway reflexively closes. Water that is breathed in is absorbed quickly, leaving mostly dry and fully functional lungs.

Though a drowned (suffocated) person goes unconscious and stops breathing, the heart continues to beat normally. During the first minutes of unconsciousness and respiratory arrest, the oxygen level will begin to drop, the heart rate will speed up in an effort to restore oxygenation, and yet the oxygen level will continue to drop. After a few more minutes, the heart rate will begin to slow down, becoming weaker in strength, and then will stop. Usually an arrhythmia such as ventricular fibrillation (irregular, nonproductive muscular twitching) starts, and then the cardiac movement slows and ceases over a few more minutes, and death ensues.

It is important to understand how death by suffocation occurs. Understanding the process of hypoxia and cardiac arrest will help you to revive a drowning victim, if it is not too late.

Once when I was on duty late at night, one of my ED nurses brought her dog to the ambulance bay. Her dog, a golden retriever, was very old and had apparently had a massive stroke. She had not moved on her own, other than a slight twitch of her left paw, in several hours, and would only utter a low moan when her owner tried to wake her. Her breathing was rapid and shallow. The nurse knew of no veterinarians who were open and asked if I would end her dog's suffering.

Chapter 15 Drowning and Near Drowning

After considering the possibilities, I realized that our phenobarbital, which is what we used at the veterinary office where I worked before medical school, was locked, along with most of the other medications, in a computerized cabinet. Taking it out required entering a patient's name, and that patient would then be billed. Earlier in the day, we had used ketamine and a paralytic agent and had discarded them in a "sharps" container. I carefully retrieved them, avoiding the used needles and scalpels. Ketamine is a powerful "sedative hypnotic" agent, which I use mostly when repairing large facial lacerations in anxious children who could never otherwise cooperate. The paralytic agent, vecuronium, is used when a patient is "intubated" with an endotracheal tube (breathing tube) to paralyze the breathing muscles and allow mechanical ventilation.

As my nurse held her old dog in her arms, I injected a triple dose of the ketamine into the dog's large leg muscle. The dog showed no sign of feeling the shot. Ketamine, given by the intramuscular route, is very well absorbed and takes about five minutes for full effect. After about five minutes, I tested the dog with a hard pinch, and there was no response. I shaved the dog's leg in the place we usually looked at the vet's office, but there were no veins visible. I could feel the dog's heart pounding beneath her thin chest wall. It felt like it was just below the surface. I inserted the needle, drawing back to ensure it was within a heart chamber, and got a flash of blood. I then injected the double dose of paralytic. Again, the dog did not show any sign of noticing the needle. I kept my hand on the dog's heart. In less than a minute, she stopped breathing. Her heart rate, already around 100 beats per minute, started to speed up. Within a minute it was in the 150-plus range. As fast as it had sped up, it began to slow, and within a minute, could no longer be felt.

In this case, the dog's breathing was stopped by the paralytic agent in the same way that drowning stops the breathing in a human victim.

If You Witness a Drowning

Knowing what to do for a victim of drowning (turning the drowning into a near drowning, in effect) relies on your understanding of the above paragraphs. If there is someone else present, immediately have them call 911. Tell him/her to "stay on the line until they hang up." If there is more than one additional person, designate someone else to help you.

Within a minute or so of unconsciousness, getting the victim's face out of the water, rough stimulation, and opening the airway is often all that is needed to restore spontaneous breathing and consciousness. The victim's heartbeat will still be fast and strong in this case.

If spontaneous breathing (gagging and coughing usually) does not begin within a few seconds, giving a rescue breath while pinching the nose may trigger spontaneous breathing. When the person vomits, roll them onto their left side while maintaining the stability of the neck. Some degree of vomiting is usual in this situation, and it is often violent and recurrent.

If a few more minutes have passed, the victim may have become hypoxic (low on oxygen), and the heart rate may have begun to slow. If this is the case, getting the face out of the water, stimulation, and clearing the airway will still be first. Gently move the head into a "neutral" position while the person is on his/her back. Be wary of the possibility of a neck injury, especially if there is a head wound (see the "Trauma" chapter).

Since there will be no immediate response in this case, the next step is to pinch the nose and give several lung-inflating breaths into the mouth while watching the chest rise. If the chest doesn't rise well, pushing the lower jaw forward while applying gentle traction to the neck will help.

The pulse should then be checked, and if it is not felt, or if it is slower than fast (slower than a hundred or so beats per minute) or weak, chest compressions should be done immediately. If you are trained in CPR, or if someone else present is, very good. If not, the idea is to compress the heart by pushing on the sternum while the person is on his or her back. Push hard enough on the lower sternum to depress the chest several inches. "Push hard and fast" is the rule. Aim for about one hundred compressions per minute. In this case we are dealing with a decrease in oxygen level, which must be remedied before spontaneous breathing and circulation can occur, and therefore hard, fast, and strong chest compressions will be needed for a minute. (A count of compressions will help—count out loud.)

If the person has not awakened and begun to cough, follow this vigorous cardiac massage with several more breaths, watching the chest rise, and then repeat. This is exhausting when done properly, and hopefully there will be someone else to help.

If more time passes without oxygen, and no pulse at all is felt, you are looking at a serious problem. Skin color changes will likely have started. Once again, start at the beginning as we discussed above, proceeding with each step until help arrives.

If there is an AED (automated external defibrillator) nearby, having this attached to the patient may allow identification of fibrillation, and a shock can often restore a normal rhythm and circulation. Often a normal rhythm is restored after the shock, but the heart is too weak to generate a pulse. In that case, more CPR will be needed, and either the heart will become more capable or will continue to slip away.

In the ER at this point, open cardiac massage is an option, since it is much more effective than closed chest CPR.

Medical Wisdom

The current trend is toward eliminating rescue breaths and proceeding straight to chest compressions. In the case of a drowning, however, rescue breaths are vital to ensure the airway is open. Just having the airway open does much to contribute to the body's oxygenation, because as oxygen within the lungs is absorbed, the lower amount of oxygen in the lungs causes an "oxygen vacuum" that draws more oxygen into the lungs. If oxygen is available, placing a high-flow face mask or high-flow nasal cannula on the patient and keeping the airway open will aid this process and can maintain oxygenation for a surprisingly long time without the act of breathing.

The drowning victim should be examined for signs of head and neck injury. Diving injuries are common. The worst cases involve serious head and neck injury, and the resultant loss of consciousness and/or paralysis is what caused the drowning. A scalp laceration with bleeding is often present. The neck injury is usually less obvious than the head injury, and all near-drowning victims should be very carefully checked for possible neck injury. Resuscitation is still the first priority, and the neck will be immobilized by the paramedics before transport to the emergency department.

In training we had a lot of fun discussing salt-water versus fresh-water drowning, and hypothermia in drowning, but these fine points will be of less use to you. Suffice it to say that the absorbed fresh or salt water can cause some electrolyte changes, and a hypothermic victim will take longer to resuscitate, requiring warming as part of the process.

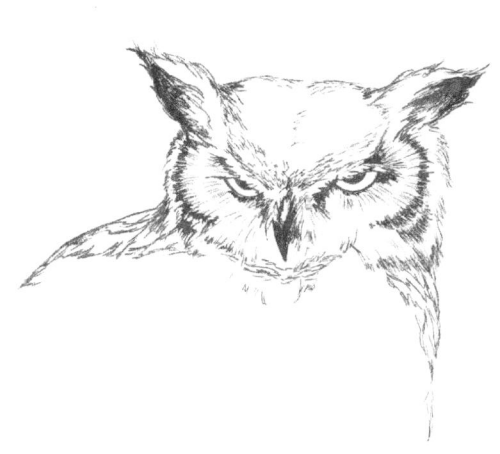

Chapter 16
Ear Pain

I think men who have a pierced ear are better prepared for marriage. They've experienced pain and bought jewelry.

—Rita Rudner

Ear pain, unless caused by injury, is generally caused either by infection or by the pressure changes of congestion. An ear infection is painful, and though it is hard to accurately estimate how much pain one-year-olds feel, if their infection is hurting as much as a similar infection in an adult, they are in a lot of pain. One of my fellow emergency physicians at the university got a middle-ear infection. Though I don't think he missed any work, we all knew of his new respect for the amount of pain the ear can cause. He talked about little else for days and was obviously very uncomfortable.

The ear is divided into three areas. The outermost ear is known as the "external ear." This part is composed of the visible ear and the ear canal to the eardrum (tympanic membrane). The eardrum, unless damaged, forms an air and watertight seal between the external and middle ear. When you pinch your nose and blow out, the pressure that you feel is air pressure in the middle ear pushing out on the eardrum from the inside. The eardrum separates the outside environment from the middle ear and inner ear. We discussed the inner ear in the "Dizziness" chapter.

External Ear Problems

The external ear sometimes becomes infected after trauma or piercings. Occasionally a piece of an earring will become lodged in the lobe, forming a small abscess, and the infection will persist until it is removed.

The ear canal is prone to an infection often referred to as "swimmer's ear." Swimmer's ear, known medically as "otitis externa" is usually caused by moisture in the canal. Dirty fresh water is likeliest to cause this infection. When I dove in the National Spearfishing Championships in Table Rock Lake, Missouri, my two teammates and I contracted this infection. We had competed in numerous saltwater contests and never had a problem, but soon realized that lake water is a different deal.

If you tug on the earlobe and the ear canal hurts, and if the ear canal is wet/oozing, it is likely you are developing swimmer's ear. Swimmer's ear is very uncomfortable, starting with a dull ache in the ear canal and progressing to sharp pains with "popping" sounds that are painful. If not treated, it progresses to a point where the canal can swell completely shut.

Eardrops are the primary treatment. I usually recommend two types of drops. The first is a mixture of antibiotic and cortisone, such as cortisporin otic suspension. This should be used for two to three days. The antibiotic will fight the infection, and the anti-inflammatory will help reduce the swelling and pain within the canal. If used too long, though, the cortisone (see the "Medications" chapter) can cause a fungal overgrowth, and the infection will continue. After the third day, the canal is less sensitive, and an acetic acid containing medication, or vinegar, can be substituted and used until the infection is resolved. In rare cases, otitis externa can progress to "malignant otitis externa," which means the infection has gone beyond the ear canal. Worsening pain and fever are likely. Eardrops are not enough in this case, and you should see a doctor promptly.

It is easier to avoid swimmers ear (otitis externa) than it is to treat it. If you will be swimming in warm lake water, mix up a solution of half white vinegar and half isopropyl alcohol, and after swimming, apply enough drops to fill each ear canal.

Middle Ear Infection

Antibiotic drops applied to the external ear will stop at the eardrum and thus are not useful for treating the commonest ear infection, which is called "otitis media."

The middle ear is just behind the eardrum, and an infection of the middle ear is common in children. Possibly, this is because the tube that drains the middle ear, the Eustachian tube, is more tortuous in youth and then straightens as the head and jaw mature. The more tortuous Eustachian tube does not drain as well, and an infection can thus develop in the middle-ear space. A middle-ear infection is painful and can result in rupture of the eardrum. If the eardrum ruptures, there will be drainage from the ear.

Some children have recurrent infections of the middle ear. Bottle feeding, and especially bottle feeding while the child is lying flat, seems to contribute. Recurrent infections should be evaluated closely and may merit a visit to the ENT specialist (otolaryngologist).

The commonest scenario is when a child gets a regular cold (viral infection) and then develops ear pain. The congestion of the cold causes swelling and decreased ear drainage, which allows the infection to occur.

A simple middle-ear infection is not considered to be a good cause (medically we say "source") of fever. Let me elaborate. If your child has a fever, the doctor will be looking for a reason for that fever. If no reason can be found, there is a possibility that a more serious, harder to find (and potentially dangerous) reason for the fever exists, such as a urinary infection or brain infection (meningitis). If the doctor sees the ear infection and stops the search there, he or she is very likely mistaken. Many children brought to the ER with ear pain and congestion do have a fever, though, and the fever is usually caused by the viral infection. As we will go over again in the infection chapter, a cold (also known as a viral syndrome) has a number of typical symptoms (e.g., cough, congestion, sore throat) and infects/affects much of the body. If an ear infection alone causes a fever, it could be a much more serious problem than a simple otitis media.

The importance of antibiotics such as amoxicillin in the treatment of otitis media is a subject of debate. Currently, most pediatricians will treat otitis media with antibiotics. In parts of Europe, the trend has been to not use antibiotics. The fact that there is debate over whether or not antibiotics are needed in otitis media indicates that antibiotics, while possibly helpful, are likely not essential in most cases. Antibiotics are also not a miracle cure for otitis, and you should expect the cold symptoms and often the fevers to continue.

Many doctors have been made to feel that parents want and expect antibiotics and will not be satisfied unless their child gets them. When you talk to your pediatrician, let him/her know that you understand the difference between viral and bacterial infection, that you realize antibiotics are useless or harmful in viral infection, and that you are going to honor his/her opinion.

Chapter 16 Ear Pain

A few things are certain about otitis media and antibiotics. If your child has serious ear pain and is kept awake and crying by the pain, antibiotics are not going to help at all for at least two or three days. It takes three doses of antibiotics to build a therapeutic blood level, and several days for the medicine to penetrate into the site of the infection. Antibiotics will do nothing to treat the cold that caused the congestion (which allowed the secondary bacterial infection to take hold). Because antibiotics will not treat the cold, they will not relieve the fever, either. Antibiotics can cause allergic reactions, diaper rash, and diarrhea, and overuse causes tougher antibiotic-resistant infections to arise.

Pain medication is needed. An anti-inflammatory such as ibuprofen will help a lot. Within twenty minutes of a full dose (ten milligrams per kilogram of body weight), the child will be much more comfortable, and the fever will usually be lower. This effect will only last for four to six hours, and more ibuprofen or Tylenol will be needed. It is safe to use both ibuprofen and Tylenol at the same time, and if the fever is high and recurrent, they can be alternated so that one or the other is always in force. A numbing medicine such as Auralgan or another anesthetic-containing solution can also be put in the ear. If it is nighttime and ibuprofen is not enough, your doctor can add Tylenol with codeine.

The latest approach to decreasing antibiotic overuse in ear infections, while also meeting parental demands, is called the "wait-and-see plan." In the wait-and-see plan, the doctor discusses with the parents the pros and cons of antibiotic use to treat ear infections and then prescribes the antibiotic prescription, to be filled and started if the child is not improving as expected. Usually the wait-and-see period is a day or two. Since the majority of the child's symptoms are caused by the cold, and since the cold usually will improve in a day or two, the antibiotics are not often needed.

Rarely, an otitis media will spread to the inner-ear structures, or mastoid bone (hard bone behind the ear), and in this rare case can cause a fever and serious problems. If this occurs, see a doctor promptly.

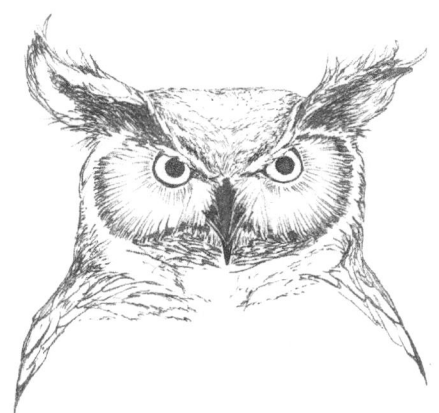

Chapter 17
Extremity Pain after Trauma

How many legs does a dog have if you call the tail a leg? Four.
Calling a tail a leg doesn't make it a leg.

—Abraham Lincoln

Injuries to the arms and legs can be as minor as a bruise or as major as an open (skin broken) fracture, serious dislocation, or amputation. There is a lot of material to cover here, but some will be in other chapters, such as the chapters on fractures and on wounds.

Although the chapter on fractures is coming up soon, I must say here that many patients think a fracture is something different than a "break." Medically speaking, a fracture and break are the same thing.

When your doctor says you have "a fracture," you have broken a bone. If, after being told that you have "fractured your hand," you ask, "Is it broken, too?" your doctor will probably smile and say, "Yes, it is both fractured and broken." A better question would be, "Which bone is fractured?" or "Is it a displaced fracture (moved out of position), or a nondisplaced fracture?"

A contusion is a blow, or impact, to a body part resulting in damage, pain, and usually swelling or bruising. Bruising is just internal bleeding that is close enough to the skin to be seen. Lots of bruising (bleeding) is deep and not visible from the surface. Pain and swelling or firmness and tenderness of tissues that would normally be soft and pain free may be the only symptoms of underlying injury.

A sprain is damage to a ligament. Ligaments are tough connective tissues that join bones to other bones. Without ligaments the bones would move back and forth upon each other and rely only on the muscles to keep them lined up. That would be a bad state of affairs. You have seen the life-sized skeleton models often used for teaching: the connections that keep them from falling apart are doing the job of ligaments. When a ligament is badly injured or disrupted, there is abnormal looseness (laxity) of the joint.

The anterior cruciate ligament (ACL), for example, keeps the big bone of the lower leg (tibia) from moving forward on the bone of the upper leg (femur). If you are a football fan, you have heard "torn ACL" many times.

To test the ACL, I have the patient sit on the edge of the bed or lying down on the back, raise the knees off the bed so they are bent. I then hold the ankle in place with my right hand and pull forward on the back of the person's calf. If the ligament is partly torn or disrupted, the lower leg will move forward and the knee joint will look visibly different as a result. If it is intact, it should move very slightly. To see if there is a slight change (partial ligamentous tear), I always test the other side as well. Some people have looser ligaments than others, and old injuries can leave more laxity. The ACL and its opposing ligament, the posterior cruciate ligament (PCL), are located within the knee joint. The PCL is tested with the same positioning as the ACL, but instead of pulling forward on the calf/tibia, I push on it.

If there is a tear in the ACL or PCL, bleeding into the joint will occur—a "joint effusion." In the "Infection" chapter, we will discuss the joint as being a closed space and thus prone to infection. Sometimes a joint effusion will become "tense" and uncomfortable. It is possible to drain some of the fluid out of the joint by using a large needle. This is called "arthrocentesis," or "tapping" a joint. The down side of arthrocentesis is that even with thorough cleansing, there is some risk of infection. The fluid also can reaccumulate. If the effusion came on after trauma, it is probably bloody and may need time for the clot to break down before it can be withdrawn through a needle. The fluid will be absorbed in time.

A strain is when a part of the body is stressed to the point that there is some degree of tearing or failure. Some fibers can tear within a muscle, causing sudden onset of pain and swelling/soreness. Sometimes the line between strain and sprain blurs.

Do I Need an X-ray?

Much of what we do for extremity trauma in the ED is aimed at determining if anything is fractured, dislocated, or otherwise seriously injured. When you hurt your arm or leg, or when your child does, the first question is whether or not you need to go to the doctor. Often it is the ER we consider, since injuries happen in an unpredictable manner and when doctor's offices are often closed. Injuries also often happen on weekends, because that is when people break from their routine and do exciting stuff—which is often a bit risky.

To help you decide whether to come in "for an X-ray," we will discuss an interesting set of rules devised in Canada in an attempt to decrease visits to the ER for ankle X-rays. The rules are called the

"Ottawa ankle rules" and are widely accepted, but not flawless. The rules definitely predict the vast majority of fractures and are definitely good enough for home use. There are a few foot fractures that can confuse things a bit, but you'll get the idea.

The commonest way to injure the ankle is with an inversion. In an inversion, the foot rolls inward, as if you were trying to see the bottom of your foot. The same sort of inversion is a great way to break the end of the smaller of the two lower leg bones, the fibula. This fracture, which is one of the commoner ones people get, can vary from a small chip of the end of the fibula to a complete break through the end of the fibula with disruption of the ligament that holds the fibula and tibia together. Thus the first ankle rule is: "If there is bone tenderness of the last six centimeters (about two inches) of the fibula, an X-ray is needed."

The second rule is the same, but applies to the end of the tibia (big bone on the inside of the ankle). A similar fracture can occur on that side. "If there is bony tenderness of the last six centimeters of the tibia, an X-ray is needed."

The third rule is different and has to do with function: "An X-ray is needed if the patient has an inability to bear weight both immediately after the injury and in the emergency department for four steps." Some athletic people can appear to be bearing weight while actually "hopping" or "shuffling," and a very severe limp should fail the rule. If a person has only a mild or moderate limp and can walk fairly well, even though there is pain, a fracture is unlikely, and an X-ray is not needed.

Because the ankle rules are successful and widely adopted, other rules were created. The Ottawa knee rules are similar. In the knee rules, the points of bony tenderness to be checked are the head of the fibula (hard bone just below the knee on the outside of the leg) and the patella (kneecap). The functional tests are "ability to flex the knee to ninety degrees," and once again, "ability to bear weight both in the emergency department and immediately after the injury for four steps."

These rules, though not exact (medicine is not exact) can help if we consider them more fully. "Bony tenderness" is mentioned repeatedly. If you can test a bone without pushing on the injured ligament and soft tissue, there is a chance you can exclude a fracture. If good function remains, there is probably no fracture.

What if your child does end up having a broken ankle and a few days pass before you bring him in? Let's say he is playing basketball and comes down hard, inverting the ankle and experiencing immediate severe pain. The coach makes him "walk it off" and he does, limping around the perimeter of the court a few times. He is given Advil and continues to play. When you see him at home, he is limping, the ankle is quite swollen, especially on the outer side, and there is bruising. You try to apply the ankle rules but are not sure about the tenderness because the swelling makes it hard to feel the fibula well. You decide against the ER visit. You call me for an opinion, and I tell you that the continued function practically guarantees that there is no fracture. Note I use the word "practically" and not "absolutely." Don't you love the way doctors do that?

A week later he is still asking for ibuprofen, so you decide to take him in for an X-ray. The X-ray shows "a nondisplaced fracture of the distal fibula." The doctor says that, yes, there is a fracture, but he is walking so well that he probably does not need a cast. He mentions several other options, including splinting and a "cam walking boot." Your son doesn't want to be slowed down, so none of those options appeal to him. You go home, and he does fine.

The above scenario is typical of minor fractures that allow good continued function. If your boy can't bear weight the day after the injury without a severe limp, and it doesn't get better with ibuprofen as the day progresses, you should probably bring him in for the X-ray. It could be that the adrenaline of competition and the coach's charisma allowed him to continue to function with a fracture. I have seen that occur only twice in almost twenty years of practice, but it can happen.

Sprains can cause a lot of pain and a lot of swelling. An ankle sprain with actual ligament damage will also be bruised. The bruising of both a fibular fracture and ankle sprain will descend to the area where the sole of the foot joins the foot, and stop at that tough fibrous junction. I used to tell patients with a serious ankle sprain that the pain could last for up to six weeks, since that was what I was told in medical school. Now I say "up to six months, possibly longer."

I suffered a serious ankle sprain with a lot of bruising about ten years ago, and the ligament still hurt a year later when stressed by rolling the ankle outward. I stepped off a trailer holding a bunch of two-by-fours in front of me and didn't see a deep, dried horse-hoof print in the clay. I never stopped walking on it, as walking seemed to decrease the pain, as it often does with sprains, and I had a long day of work ahead. It was so severely bruised three days later (OK, I had to show off!) that one of my senior residents talked me into getting an X-ray, which turned out normal. The coach is often right to say, "Walk it off."

Intoxication and Pain

A high level of alcohol at the time of the injury can hide a fracture. Once I treated a man at the trauma center who had fallen down the stairs in front of a downtown bar. The friend who brought him in said he had the hand rail in his right hand, but it swung him around so he went down backward, tangling in the railing and dumping onto the concrete walk, hitting his head. He had an obvious lump on his forehead with an abrasion. I examined him head to toe in a gown and noted a few other minor abrasions and a mild swelling of the right knee. I could move the knee well without apparent pain. Partially because of his intoxication, he was placed on a rigid backboard with a cervical collar. After his neck X-rays and head CT came back negative (for fractures), we "cleared" him from the board, leaving the cervical collar on, as was our policy with intoxicated patients. He wanted to go to the bathroom and refused to use a urinal at the bedside. His speech was slurred.

At about that time, one of my residents walked up and said, "Guess his BAL (blood alcohol level)." I carefully recalled his actions, since my pride was on the line. I explained to the resident that he seemed to be a "rather experienced drinker" but yet appeared quite intoxicated. I hazarded a guess at 400. He was 385. That made him roughly four times the legally drunk level. The resident said, "Not bad!" In my head I calculated how long we would need to watch him to get him below .08. Legally drunk in California is .08. A BAL of .10, which we refer to as 100, means that one-tenth of a percent of a person's blood and body fluid is alcohol. Four hundred and fifty is very high (.450) and would render a less-experienced drinker unconscious.

Most toxic chemicals have what is called a "lethal dose 50," or LD50. The LD50 is the level where, without medical treatment, half of the people with that level will die. The LD50 for ethyl alcohol is 500, or .50. I have seen only half a dozen or so patients brought in over 500, and none of them died, but I did need to intubate several (breathing tube in trachea) and support them.

Anyway, back to the story. I calculated that since the average drinker metabolizes alcohol at about .025 per hour, if we wanted to keep him until he was down to .08, we'd be sitting on him for about twelve hours. Since I was working a twelve-hour shift, I would get to see much of it. He still wanted to go to the bathroom and was trying to lower the bed rail. Failing that, he began scooting off the end of the bed. I walked over and spoke to him again about the urinal. He was having none of that, and stood up. He walked to the bathroom with his nurse in tow. He had no apparent limp and was surprisingly stable on his feet. He had a broad-based gait, but otherwise did well. Before one of us could lower the rail, he walked back from the bathroom, crawled from the end of the bed to the head on his knees, and flopped down. I hooked him to a pulse oximeter with an alarm.

He maintained his oxygen saturation while snoring loudly for about four hours. After four hours he repeated the trip to the bathroom, this time needing no nurse to help. I watched him go, and he walked well, but with a slight limp on the right leg that had not been present the previous time. The resident had not noticed the knee swelling, and I discussed it with him at this time. By now the BAL would probably be around .250, because a truly experienced drinker's liver can metabolize alcohol faster than normal. My resident examined the knee when the patient returned. The ligaments were stable, but the effusion had increased in size. We ordered an X-ray. The X-ray took longer than usual, which in the crowded university ED is pretty long. There were some serious trauma cases, which delayed everything as well.

About four hours later, the patient needed to go to the bathroom again. He swung out of bed, but then just stood there. He tried to take a step, said something along the lines of, "God XXXX my XXXXXXX knee hurts!" He chose to use the urinal at his bedside and got back in bed. By now his alcohol level was likely around 130 or so, a bit less than twice legally drunk. The X-ray showed a "tibial plateau fracture." A tibial plateau fracture is a very painful fracture involving the weight-bearing surface of the tibia at the knee. No normal person could have walked on that fracture, and neither could he when some of the alcohol was metabolized.

Immobilization?

Deciding whether to immobilize an extremity injury depends on several factors. Immobilization can be done solely for comfort if moving the injury causes more pain. Even if nothing is actually torn or fractured, this can help for a few days and may be needed. Fractures and major ligament injuries should be immobilized, of course. If there is no structural damage, continued movement can decrease pain, prevent the swelling that would soon cause pain, and speed recovery. As the coach says, "Walk it off."

Some joints don't handle long-term immobilization very well. For example, the elbow tends to become stiff and if immobilized in a bent position for more than a few weeks and will require some rehabilitation to restore normal movement. Fingers tend to stiffen into the bent position and should thus be splinted straight. The joint where the finger joins the hand, known as the metacarpophalangeal joint (knuckle) tends to stiffen in the straightened position, making it tough to form a fist. If that joint needs to be immobilized it should be in a bent position, rather than straight. To demonstrate the proper positions of immobilization for the hand, form an "L" with the fingers and hand by keeping the fingers straight/extended and bending the knuckles. You have no doubt seen that position in casts before, or some attempt at achieving it, at least.

An obvious deformity of an extremity means a substantial injury of some sort and should be immobilized. If medical attention will not be available soon, a deformed bone may need to be straightened or a joint relocated. We will discuss some of those techniques in the "Fractures and Dislocations" chapter.

Applying ice to a recent injury for the first day is generally recommended. The icing can help reduce pain and decrease swelling. After the first day, warmth may help to increase circulation, loosen up a stiffened injury, and decrease pain with movement. Sometimes massage can be good for a painful muscle strain or spasm. For a spasm, massage can be good right away, as can an injection of lidocaine, especially if there is a palpable "trigger point." A muscle tear, though, may be too tender and may need to recover first.

Pain after a Motor Vehicle Collision

In the ER we see a lot of patients one to three days after a motor-vehicle collision. At the time of the collision, the patient was "fine." As time passed, things started to hurt. The usual complaints are neck and back pain, but often there are extremity injuries as well. I have x-rayed thousands of these people, and in only two cases did I find a fracture. In both cases, a lot of alcohol was involved, obscuring the injury initially. It is normal to have some aches and pains hours to days after a substantial jolt, but a fracture is a real attention grabber and will be noticed immediately.

As the years have gone by I have become increasingly selective about X-rays in the "one to three days after the accident" group. Initially I x-rayed pretty much everyone. Then I changed my practice to asking a lot of questions, doing a good exam as usual, and then posing the question: "So of all things, what hurts the very worst?" or "Which injury caused you to come to the ER?" I would then x-ray that particular part. When it came back negative, I would have already given pain medicine. If the patient was not reassured and was still worried about the other painful areas, I would order more X-rays. Since I still was finding no fractures, I further refined my practice to add a functional test: if the person can use the painful body part normally, I offer reassurance after examining for bony tenderness, and discuss care, pain control, and recovery, skipping the X-ray in most cases.

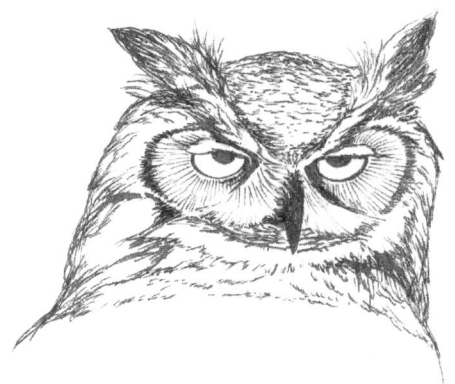

Chapter 18
Extremity Pain without Trauma

Be temperate in wine, in eating, girls, and cloth or the gout will
seize you and plague you both.

—*Benjamin Franklin*

In the "Trauma" chapter, we will cover some aspects of arm and leg injury, and in the "Fractures and Dislocations" chapter, we will cover broken bones in particular. The focus of this chapter is pain in the arms or legs that is not associated with an injury.

Sometimes pain in an extremity is caused by "overuse," and in that case, we are dealing with a sort of trauma, though it is the accumulated trauma of many small injuries.

You may ask, "What would an emergency physician know about problems like this?" Well, pain is pain, and I treat these problems in the ER on most if not every shift.

Every tissue type can be affected by overuse, and though good hearty use is good for the body, there comes a point when either the wear and tear causes more damage than can be repaired, or the body begins to perceive the inflammation as chronic, rather than an injury. Usually, the body can repair damage quickly and completely, but sometimes the damage occurs faster than repair can occur. Alternately, the damage can cause scarring, which can compress sensitive structures.

Nerve Entrapment /Impingement

If the scarring causes pressure on a nerve that is either surrounded or pinned against an unyielding structure, nerve entrapment/impingement problems can occur. These problems can then be aggravated by overuse. Carpal tunnel syndrome is an example of such a problem. In carpal tunnel syndrome, the median nerve is compressed where it enters the hand through a narrow place in the wrist called...you guessed it, the carpal tunnel. Repeated movement of the wrist can cause inflammation, swelling, and scarring in this narrow space, which then causes compression of the nerve. The median nerve supplies sensation to the thumb, index, and middle fingers, as well as power to the muscles of the hand in that area. As the nerve is irritated and compressed numbness and tingling are felt, and later weakness is experienced in those fingers.

Resting the wrist and avoiding flexion, which causes the worst compression, is often a successful treatment. The first wise step is to wear a wrist splint at night. Even though people don't know it, it is natural to flex the wrists when asleep. Because of this prolonged flexion, the pain and numbness are often worse in the morning. Surgical decompression is sometimes needed eventually, and decompression of the median nerve at the carpal tunnel is a very common procedure for hand specialists.

There are so many impingement and compression syndromes that it would be tedious to cover them all. Instead, we will continue to discuss some of the commoner ones, and the knowledge you gain will help you understand other similar conditions.

An example of a nerve impingement is often seen in the lower back. Sciatica is the compression of the components of or of the sciatic nerve itself. We discussed Sciatica in the "Back Pain" chapter. The sciatic nerve emerges from the lowest lumbar and upper sacral levels of the spinal cord. When this nerve is irritated, pain, numbness, or other strange sensations go down the back of the leg, continuing sometimes along the nerve's entire route. The nerve supplies sensation to the lateral (outside) side of the lower leg, and to the top of the foot. The nerve also powers the muscles at the front of the lower leg, which allow "dorsiflexion" (lifting up) of the foot and toes.

When a disc bulge or muscle spasm (see "Back Pain" chapter) presses on the nerve lightly, a shooting pain or numbness will often occur. With prolonged or heavier pressure, the ability of the nerve to function may be impaired, and if this occurs, weakness of dorsiflexion can result. This is called foot drop and is a serious sign. As we discussed in the back pain chapter, if a nerve loses motor function, it may be losing the battle against that bulge, scar, or spasm. Prompt treatment is needed.

I suffered from sciatica for about a year, and one of the sensations I experienced was unique. I would be standing there at work, and I could swear someone threw a bucket of hot water on the outside of my right lower leg! The first few times it happened, I spun and looked accusingly to the right, ready to curse someone for a silly prank. Two of my nurses were frequently up to such pranks and had been known to squirt warm water on people with syringes, so I thought of them instantly. But it wasn't them. Any sensation that a nerve can experience can be duplicated by stimulation of (pressure on) that nerve!

It is important to differentiate between pain, which prevents full demonstration of strength, and the actual lack of strength. It is the actual lack of strength that is more concerning.

The nerves that supply sensation and power to the arms exit the spinal cord in the neck. Recurrent shooting pains to the arms when the neck moves is suspicious for a cervical (neck) impingement problem. Arm weakness caused by the nerves of the neck has the same significance as that of the lower back. A spinal MRI will be needed for diagnosis, and if a problem that corresponds to the symptom is seen on MRI, surgical treatment can have excellent results.

The sacral (below the lowest low back) nerves are responsible for sensation to the "saddle" area (roughly the part that contacts the horse when riding). These nerves are also responsible for some motor function, though it is of a different sort than leg and arm movement. Failure of these nerves causes problems in bowel, bladder, and sexual function. Bowel and bladder function are the most obvious failures, but sometimes the urinary failure can be inability to urinate (urinary retention), and that can result in a delay of diagnosis.

Tendonitis

Tendons can become painful from overuse or repeated stresses. A common example of a tendon irritation occurs with repeated dorsiflexion (cocking up) of the wrist. Kayakers with offset paddles can get this problem, and I have also seen it in bricklayers and chefs. This particular tendonitis (inflammation of the tendon) is called De Quervain's tenosynovitis and occurs on the radial (thumb) side of the wrist.

Tendons have a slippery lubricant that allows them to slide through a tube called a tendon sheath. Repeatedly sliding through the sheath under tension depletes this lubricant's effectiveness and causes loss of the smooth sliding. When felt during movement, the normally slippery-smooth feeling is replaced by a dry, "ratchety" sensation, which causes injury, swelling, and pain.

Another common tendonitis occurs at the kneecap (patella).

Tendonitis is treated by rest, and an anti-inflammatory such as ibuprofen will help. Given a few weeks (in bad cases), the tendon and sheath will heal their abraded surfaces, and the lubricant will once again be effective.

Sometimes these overuse-type injuries can be very persistent. It is not unusual for an epicondylitis (tennis elbow) to last for a bit over a year! It is obviously important to keep using the painful elbow, in the case of epicondylitis, since long-term immobilization will cause stiffness and weakness. Ibuprofen will help a lot, but only for about eight hours at best, so you will need repeated doses.

Blood Vessel Problems

Vascular (blood vessel) problems can cause pain in the arms or legs. The problems caused by veins and arteries are very different, and we will discuss both.

Probably the commonest and most dangerous problem with veins is clotting. Since the blood flows slower in veins, the blood can clot, blocking the vein partially or completely. Serious clots occur most commonly in the legs, and the deep veins of the legs are the source of this problem.

When a superficial vein clots, a painful spot visible and easily palpable beneath the skin occurs. This is called a "superficial phlebitis." Though irritating, it is not dangerous. A superficial clot usually seems to occur in the calf or behind the knee.

Though the location of origin is similar for a deep leg-vein clot, the problem is much more serious. Clotting starts in the deep vein of the calf and will then extend upward to the thigh and even into the deep veins of the abdomen. Signs of this problem include a dull ache in the calf that worsens with foot movement or rubbing the area, swelling of the calf on the affected side, prominent veins of the foot and lower leg, and possibly discoloration of the lower leg.

The most dangerous thing about this type of clot is that it can break off and ride the flow of blood to the heart. The clot is then pumped from the heart into the lung. At this point the clot is called a "pulmonary (lung) embolus." Some chest pain may be felt, but if the clot is toward the center of the lung, the pain is usually minimal. If the clot is small, it may not even be noticed, but if it is big, it can block enough blood flow to cause shortness of breath, chest pain, and syncope (passing out). At worst a big clot can cause sudden death.

A number of things create a risk for deep venous clots, and understanding something about how the blood vessels work will help you to both avoid this problem and to recognize it early if it does occur.

When a person sits in a chair and the legs are dependent and immobile, the blood will fill the veins to capacity. Swelling of the legs occurs, since the veins and capillaries (smallest vessels which bridge the gap between the smallest arteries and smallest veins) are not watertight, but are actually permeable to the fluid component of the blood. Gas and fluid/nutrient exchange occurs across the vessel walls. When the pressure on the venous side is unusually high, such as when a clot is obstructing the return of blood toward the heart, the amount of fluid exiting exceeds the amount reentering, and swelling occurs. The veins run through and between the leg muscles, so when the leg muscles contract, the blood is pushed along through the veins. Since the veins have valves that prevent backflow, the blood is pushed toward the heart.

When walking or standing, the leg muscles are constantly relaxing and contracting, and the blood keeps moving. When a person is immobile, the pooled blood is at the highest risk of clotting. Periods of immobility are a risk factor for blood clots of the legs. I have seen patients with clots after airplane flights and long drives.

A period of bed rest in the hospital is a very serious risk, and patients who are hospitalized will usually be treated with either blood thinners or stockings/inflating pants to mimic the "leg muscle pump."

Chapter 18 Extremity Pain without Trauma

Deep venous thrombosis (DVT) accounts for about 200,000 deaths annually and is the leading cause of preventable in-hospital death. If you or a loved one is hospitalized, ensure that the subject of blood-clot risk is addressed.

A Case of DVT

When I was a resident, I saw a young Hispanic woman in her eighth month of pregnancy who was complaining of a cough and shortness of breath. One of my interns had seen her first, as is customary, and presented the patient to me, explaining that he felt her shortness of breath and cough were caused either by a cold or by the fact that her distended uterus was pressing on her diaphragm. He explained that her oxygenation was a bit decreased, at 95 percent (normal for a young nonsmoker is 98–100 percent), but that he felt her cough accounted for that. It sounded good to me, and I went in to see her.

She was looking a bit short of breath, but had good color. Her breath sounds were clear. I pulled the sheets down and palpated her uterus, which was appropriate for eight months. Her legs were covered by the sheets. Sometimes in pregnancy the legs swell a bit, and after reassuring her, I gave her calves a squeeze (through the sheets as I was preparing to leave the room) to check for the extent of that swelling. She said, "Aiyy!" and drew her right leg back. I pulled up the sheet and saw an ace wrap on her right calf. I asked in Spanish and she told me it had started hurting a week ago, and she had been using the wrap for the pain. She had not mentioned the leg pain to my intern. Ultrasound showed that the pain was caused by a deep venous thrombosis. That was a close call! Pregnancy is a risk factor for DVT.

Some other risk factors for blood clotting include injury to the extremity, cancer, birth control or other hormone use, smoking, and obesity. Rarely a blood clot can form in the arm. I have seen two of these, but have talked to many doctors who have never seen one. In both cases there was visible swelling of the arm veins and a dull, aching discomfort similar to that felt in the leg.

An arterial obstruction or decrease in flow to an arm or leg is much more painful than a venous obstruction. A decrease in arterial flow is commonly seen in patients who have a heavy smoking history. Pain occurs when demand exceeds blood supply, and this pain is called claudication. Insufficient arterial flow will result in a reproducible degree of pain with exertion of the affected muscles. Vascular surgeons talk about claudication in terms of how many blocks of walking it takes for the pain to come. You may have felt this sort of burning, aching pain if your ski boots or ice skates were too tight.

Venous obstruction causes a darkening or reddening of the extremity, whereas arterial obstruction causes pallor. "Venous insufficiency" means the veins are not flowing as well as they should. Venous insufficiency causes swelling, and over time the swelling and decreased circulation that results from that swelling can cause skin problems. The skin problems from venous obstruction or insufficiency most often occur on the lower, inner calf. This area is known as the "gaiter" region, since it is part of the leg used to control the horse (or mule!) by applying pressure to his sides. Skin breakdown and ulcers (slow or nonhealing erosions) are typical when venous "return" is compromised.

Arterial flow problems, as you would expect, first cause pain and pallor at the ends of the toes and fingers. These places are farthest from the source of the pressure.

Extremity pain can come from infection, and sometimes there is no apparent reason for the infection. The commonest infection of this sort is cellulitis, an infection of the skin. The commonest place for this to occur is the shin area, or calf. Painful redness and heat starts and then spreads. Antibiotics are very effective for cellulitis. If the cellulitis hardens and results in an abscess (boil), however, antibiotics are not likely to help much. We will talk about why antibiotics work so well in cellulitis and so poorly in the presence of an abscess, in the chapter on infection.

Joint Pain

Joint pain can have many causes. Arthritis is swelling and inflammation of a joint. The inevitable type of arthritis is called osteoarthritis. Osteoarthritis (joints with some wear on them) comes to all of us with getting older, but can start early in a joint that is misused or injured. In osteoarthritis, when a person gets up in the morning, the joints are stiff and sore. After a few minutes of moving around, though, things loosen up, and walking becomes less uncomfortable. The aching will tend to return after a period of immobility, such as a nap, but then go away again. Rheumatoid arthritis, on the other hand, gets better with rest and worse as the day goes on. My father (the orthopedist) said, "The patient with osteoarthritis can be found on the golf course, while the patient with rheumatoid arthritis is curled up in front of the TV."

Osteoarthritis affects most people to some extent in their forties and gets worse from there. My fishing buddy Jerry McGuiness (who has been sixty-nine for a long time) said once, "If you wake up after fifty and something doesn't hurt, you probably died and went to heaven during the night." Jerry is usually out on his boat fishing when I try to find him.

The best medications for osteoarthritis are the nonsteroidal anti-inflammatory medications such as ibuprofen and aspirin. It would be great if these medications actually stopped inflammation, but they don't actually do much to stop things from swelling up. They do relieve the pain that is associated with swelling, though, and they are not addictive. Aspirin has other beneficial effects for people over fifty years old, which include decreasing the chance of thrombotic stroke

(stroke caused by a blood clot) and decreasing heart attacks caused by blood clots.

For years I heard that a person should not take aspirin with other nonsteroidals, and people are often led to believe that there is an interaction. There is no particular interaction, but caution should be used because they are additive. If aspirin alone is not enough for pain relief, adding ibuprofen, for example, without decreasing the aspirin dose to compensate, will be hard on the stomach. If aspirin alone is not enough, cutting back to an aspirin a day and using a slightly decreased dose of another anti-inflammatory is an option.

Eating these large pills with some food may help ease their impact on the stomach, but the primary way that anti-inflammatory pain medications hurt the stomach is not by direct contact. The stomach and esophagus are normally protected from stomach acid by protective mechanisms that are partially removed by the anti-inflammatory effect. The stomach acid then can damage the stomach. Even injections and intravenous nonsteroidal anti-inflammatories have the potential to result in stomach pain and damage. Acid-stopping medications such as Zantac can help decrease this damage, and in some cases your doctor may recommend this approach. It is a good idea to ask your doctor about the best course of action when it comes to "taking medicines, so that you can take more medicines," though, as things can start to get complicated!

Opiates and other addictive medications should be used with caution in arthritis, since there is no clear end point to the pain. Opiates are great for a broken bone or other acute injury that is expected to hurt for hours or days, but if used for more than a few weeks, they cause problems.

Steroid/anesthetic mixtures can be injected into a joint and give relief from osteoarthritis, but also, after repeated injections, cause further joint problems. Most orthopedists will limit a particular joint to a certain number of injections.

Chapter 18 Extremity Pain without Trauma

Joint replacement is an option when a joint is worn out, and pain medications are no longer enough. Most joint replacement can be done under spinal or regional anesthesia, so the risks are minimal.

If you are heading for a knee replacement, realize that the best plan is to "walk in and walk out." Patients who are active when the replacement is done do much better than those who have been sidelined by the pain.

Nothing substitutes for weight-bearing exercise (walking). The human body is a very efficient machine, and if it doesn't need to walk, it will quickly allow those walking muscles to grow small and soft and the leg bones to grow thin and weak. As we discussed in the "Diet and Exercise" chapter, small soft muscles use a lot less energy than big firm ones, and the human body does not waste energy. Small soft leg muscles will not help you recover from a joint replacement!

The best bet is to use a combination of non-narcotic pain medications, walking, and weight training during the months before the replacement to optimize strength and fitness. After the replacement you will be able to get back to the level of fitness you achieved before surgery and should be able to dispense with the pain medication after recovery from the postsurgical pain.

Rheumatoid arthritis is a serious, recurrent joint inflammation that can eventually cause joint destruction and deformity. Rheumatoid arthritis can be diagnosed by a blood test and should be managed by a rheumatologist.

Gouty arthritis is an acute and highly painful inflammation of a particular joint, and often the joint at the base of the big toe is affected. Benjamin Franklin was plagued by this problem. The classic picture of gouty arthritis is a moderately obese, middle-aged man in a recliner with an elevated, reddened, throbbing big toe. The joint at the base of the big toe is problematic and chronically painful in many people, not just those with gout. The pain in this joint is usually mild and tolerable, but in an attack of gout, it becomes much more severe, and the joint becomes red and swollen.

Gout is caused by a high level of uric acid, which then crystallizes in a joint. Other joints can be affected, and sometimes an acute attack will follow a mild trauma to the joint. Anti-inflammatory medications such as ibuprofen will relieve much of the pain, and there are prescription medications to lower the uric acid level, which over time can prevent further attacks.

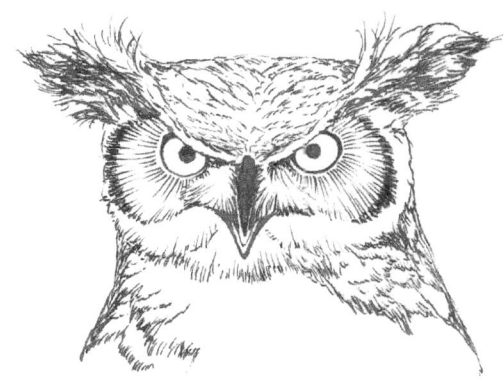

Chapter 19
Eye Emergencies

Don't run with that pencil, you could put an eye out.

—my mother, Ruth

Eye emergencies can be divided into those that occur as a result of trauma and those that arise spontaneously. The eye is very sensitive, and trauma is hard to miss in most cases. The distinction can blur at times, though, when an eye infection occurs. Once "pinkeye" has started, it can feel like there is something in the eye. It is important to make it clear if there was a particular moment/incident when something got in the eye or when the eye was injured. Once the smooth, slippery surface of the eye is scratched off or removed by the erosive effect of infection, it feels as if there is something in the eye, even though there is not.

Vision is "the vital sign" of the eye. Testing visual acuity is part of every evaluation for an eye problem and will usually be done by the triage nurse or the ED nurse or tech before you are seen by the doctor. If there is a decrease in vision not caused by watering or mucus (goop), the problem is much more serious and will likely require an ophthalmologist.

Pinkeye

Conjunctivitis, commonly called "pinkeye," is the commonest eye infection. In conjunctivitis, both the globe and lids are reddened, and there is often exudate (mucus/goop). Conjunctivitis can be caused by a virus, which is often the case in children with a cold, or by a bacterial infection. It is hard, if not impossible, to differentiate between the two, so most doctors will err toward treatment with antibiotic eye drops or ointment. If the infection is bacterial, the antibiotic is a "miracle cure," and the eye will be better within a few doses. If the infection is viral, the antibiotic will have no effect. A viral conjunctivitis will go away on its own, as will the rest of the viral infection (cold).

Some antibiotics can cause eye irritation with continued use. If the eye initially improves and then, after a few days, begins to redden again, this may be the case. This occurs frequently with an antibiotic called Gentamycin, and I have seen so many people come to the ER for eye pain and redness after being given that drug that I no longer use it for eye infections.

Eye Injury

If the surface of the eye is injured, especially the clear part (cornea), pain and the feeling that "something is in there" occurs. The cornea is very sensitive. Staining the eye with a small amount of dye will demonstrate any defect (rough spot) in the normally slick surface of the eye. Before the dye is placed, your doctor will instill some topical anesthetic drops. If the injury is to the eye surface, these drops should promptly give a lot of relief. A corneal injury will need to be treated with pain medications after you are sent home and also usually antibiotics.

The eye heals fast, and unless an infection occurs, it should feel a lot better within twenty-four hours. If the injured area becomes white and is visible to the naked eye without dye staining, there is a serious problem. This is an infection called a "corneal ulcer" and will require an ophthalmologist in most cases.

Contact-lens wearers should switch to glasses while an injury or infection heals. Patching the eye was common practice years ago, but is now rarely done. The idea was to protect the eye, but the eye still moves, rubbing against the lid, unless the other eye is patched as well.

Loss of Vision/Decreased Vision

Sudden loss of vision is very serious and should result in a prompt trip to the ED or ophthalmologist. In general, if the visual loss is confined to one eye, the ophthalmologist is the best bet. You should be seen right away. If the visual loss (without trauma) affects both eyes, the problem could be in the brain, and the ED, where a CT scan or MRI can be done, will likely be your best place to go.

Most people have some "floaters." Floaters are small, moving, often filamentous objects that are seen when one looks at a light-colored background or at the sky. Floaters are caused by wrinkles, vessels, or other deposits within the jelly (vitreous) of the eyeball. These become more common with age and are harmless, but can be annoying. A sudden change in floaters, or a big, flashing "floater" can be the sign of a serious retinal problem known as "retinal detachment" and needs emergent ophthalmologic evaluation.

Any time the eyeball (globe) is punctured, immediate medical attention is mandatory. So walk with that pencil!

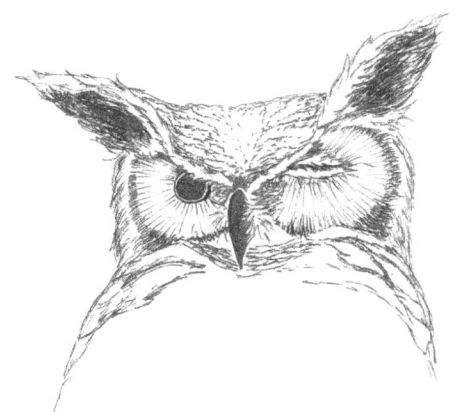

Chapter 20
Fever

My temperature runs a couple of degrees high, around a hundred.
I don't mind. It's the engine or something.

—Matty in the movie *Body Heat*

Fever is not a disease itself, but a response of the body to a disease or problem. Usually a fever occurs in response to infection, but a fever can also arise after injury or a blood clot, and it can occasionally be caused by a medication or drugs.

When a fever occurs in response to infection, it is a cause of discomfort but very rarely of any danger.

Fever Can Have a Purpose

Fever is an attempt by the body to kill the infection. This seems like a bad plan, since we don't often see good results from a fever, but a fever can indeed help to eradicate some infections. Dr. Julius Warner-Jauregg won the Nobel Prize in Medicine in 1927 by discovering that a fever could help to treat dementia paralytica, which is caused by syphilis.

Currently, syphilis is known as an uncommon sexually transmitted disease that is easily cured with antibiotics, but before antibiotics, mental institutions were packed with people, mostly between twenty and forty years old, who were suffering from this progressive, incurable, and eventually deadly disease. Dr. Jauregg needed to find an infection that would cause high, intermittent fevers but not itself kill the patient. Some infections caused a fever, but not high enough or long-lasting enough. One strain of malaria caused great fevers, but unfortunately killed some patients! Eventually, Dr. Jauregg settled on one of the less-deadly forms of malaria. Malaria causes a high, relapsing fever, which knocked down the far more debilitating disease of syphilis. This "treatment," initially argued by some to be inhumane, allowed thousands of people who would have otherwise been doomed to dementia, paralysis, and certain death, to lead productive lives. Malaria was used to cause fever as an effective syphilis treatment as recently as the early 1950s.

Some people are more prone to develop fevers than others. When a whole family catches a cold, often several members will have fevers, and others will not. Children are generally likelier to develop a noticeable fever with a given cold than are adults.

Fever in Children

In children less than three months old, and especially under two months of age, fever is a very serious symptom. Any child under two months of age with a fever should promptly be seen by a doctor.

Chapter 20 Fever

We will discuss this again in more detail in the "Pediatric Problems" chapter.

Children often have fevers, and a fever is one of the commonest reasons for a parent to bring their child to the ER. If the child is over three months of age, is acting normally, is adequately hydrated, and is well appearing, the nurse in my ER is allowed (protocol) to give either Tylenol or ibuprofen for the fever before I see the patient. I personally think that Tylenol works better for children under one year of age, whereas ibuprofen (Motrin, Advil) works better for older children. More often than not, if it takes me more than fifteen minutes to see the child, they are looking "as good as new" by the time I get there. Tylenol or ibuprofen, when given in the recommended dose, will usually lower the fever by two or three degrees Fahrenheit. If the temperature is 104, ibuprofen will usually get it down to 101 or 102, but usually not to the normal oral temperature of 98.6. At a temp of 100 or so, the child is much more playful, curious, and content than at 103 or 104.

It should be noted that temperatures vary a bit according to how and when they are taken. As stated above, the normal oral temperature is 98.6 Fahrenheit, which equals 37 degrees centigrade/Celsius. The normal rectal temperature is a bit higher, averaging around 99.0. For speed and ease when you arrive at the ER, your or your child's temperature may be taken by a skin probe or a tympanic membrane (ear) probe. Both of these tend to underestimate the temperature by half a degree or so, but are still useful for detecting a fever. If a skin probe says 99.5, it is worth repeating the measurement with an oral or rectal probe, especially if the information is critical, as in the case of a child less than three months old.

It is worth reviewing that in children, an ear infection is not considered a source of fever. What usually happens is that a cold (viral infection/viral syndrome) causes a fever, cough, sore throat, and congestion. The congestion then decreases the drainage from the middle ear by inflaming the Eustachian tube, through which fluid usually exits the middle ear. The fluid then becomes "stagnant," and inflammation of the middle ear occurs. We went over this in the ear chapter, but it is such a common problem in children that it merits further discussion. The ear is a small area, and in order to cause a fever, the infection would need to spread beyond the middle ear, at which point it becomes a much more serious problem. An isolated ear infection (without an accompanying cold) that causes a fever is a very serious problem until definitively proven otherwise.

Febrile seizures can occur in children up to five years old. A febrile seizure is a full-body seizure that can last for up to five minutes and causes no lasting damage. Up to 4 percent of children are prone to a seizure when their temperature rises.

Sometimes parents will bring in their child and complain that when they give the ibuprofen, the fever goes away, but it returns about four hours later. That is a normal occurrence. Ibuprofen and Tylenol do nothing to cure the infection, and if the infection is still causing the fever, it will return when the medication wears off, which is in about four to six hours. At that time, another dose will be needed. Parents who are concerned that the fever will return can give Tylenol alternating with ibuprofen, one or the other, every two hours. If a child is prone to febrile seizures, this may be a good practice.

Parents are often concerned that a high fever will cause brain damage. This is a myth. Fevers caused by infection are mostly beneficial, since they turn on the immune system and can create a hostile environment for the infection, which, being a human infection, does best at normal human body temperature (remember the 1927 Nobel Prize!). Body temperatures over 108 degrees (do not confuse this with 100.8 degrees) can damage the brain, but temperatures this high are not caused by the body normally and only result from an environmental problem, such as being stuck in a closed car on a hot day or passing out in a sauna when really drunk. Heat stroke, which occurs when a hot, dehydrated person stops sweating, is another way the temperature can rise. If a person with heat stroke remains in the direct sun, the body temperature can rise to a dangerous level.

Fever in the Elderly

Probably the commonest source of fever and confusion in the elderly patient with no obvious cause is a urinary-tract infection. When I first saw a case of this as a medical student, I thought, "Wow, that is weird; I'll probably never see that again," but I sure was wrong. Never does a month go by when I fail to see a worried son or daughter bring his or her elderly parent to the ER in a complete state of confusion. Rarely did they ever complain of the pain with urination or the frequency of urination that younger patients notice. When grandma or grandpa gets a fever without cold symptoms, becomes weaker than usual, is less mobile or self-reliant, becomes confused, or falls, a urine infection is high on the list of possibilities. Untreated, a urinary-tract infection can progress to an infection of the bloodstream (sepsis) and can result in death. We will talk more about urinary-tract infections in the "Urinary Problems" chapter.

Chills are associated with a release of bacteria/infectious particles into the blood. Everyone who has a fever will feel cold, but a "shaking chill" is different. Bacterial pneumonia is probably the number one cause of an actual chill, which is an uncontrollable shaking episode, usually lasting from seconds to minutes. A urinary-tract infection that has progressed to the kidneys will also cause chills when the bacterial infection moves from the urine to the blood.

Pneumonia can be more subtle in the elderly, and if the urine is normal, the lungs are the next (hidden) place to look.

We will discuss fever further in other chapters, including the "Infection" and "Shortness of Breath" chapters.

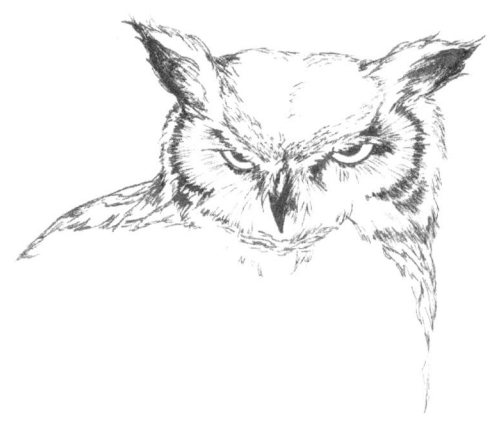

Chapter 21
Fractures and Dislocations

I will respect the privacy of my patients, for their problems are not disclosed to me that the world may know. Most especially must I tread with care in matters of life and death. If it is given to me to save a life, all thanks. But it may also be within my power to take a life; this awesome responsibility must be faced with great humbleness and awareness of my own frailty. Above all, I must not play at God.

—from a modern version of the Hippocratic Oath, by Dr. Louis Lasagna, 1964

In the chapter on extremity pain after trauma, we noted that in medical lingo a broken bone is called a "fracture." In case you skipped to this chapter, please don't ask your physician, "Is it broken, too?"

when you're told you have a fracture. You will know so much more about fractures soon that you will have a lot of other important questions to ask. All of these questions will make you seem medically wise, rather than naïve. When your doctor realizes you have some knowledge, he or she will be irresistibly tempted to add to that base of knowledge, and you will receive better care.

Bone Can Come…Bone Can Go

Bones are a complex and interesting structure. The outside of the bone is hard and shiny/smooth, but the inside is rough and composed of spaces linked by a honeycomb-like design where there are many cells and quite a bit of blood flow. The bones are thus very much alive, rather than being an unchanging framework. Bones thicken and strengthen as needed to do their job. A boxer will have thick strong bones in his arms, which have developed from the repeated stressful impacts as he works out on the bag. A runner has a higher bone density in his/her legs than a nonrunner. These changes occur over a period of months and years and require consistently repeated stress.

Lack of use has the opposite effect on bone strength (density). When a fractured arm or leg is put in a cast, the bone density (and muscle strength) decreases measurably as the weeks pass. Some decrease in bone density occurs with age. This is partly due to the normal aging process and partially due to the lowered activity level of (most) older people. If a bone is no longer needed, it will try to "go away." The body is an amazingly efficient machine and does not waste much energy.

When a cast is placed, the goal is not complete immobilization. If the fractured bone is completely immobilized, it will heal very slowly, if at all! I suppose the body figures that if no bony strength is needed at that location, why waste perfectly good calcium and energy rebuilding the bone? This is why once the initial pain begins to decrease, a cast is often modified to allow some use of the extremity, and the patient is told to "put some weight on it if you can without too much pain."

Every bone in the body turns over completely about every five years. Calcium is constantly leaving the bones, and new calcium being laid down. If you are worried about bone density, you can easily shift the balance in your favor and see higher bone strength as the result. I punch a heavy bag in the garage several times a week not because I am a boxer, but because I don't want to break an arm when I fall off my mule, which happens on occasion. I also trot my mules on the road regularly. The impact is bound to make their leg bones stronger.

Sometimes a fracture is obvious, and sometimes it is very subtle. This mostly depends on the type of fracture.

Types of Fractures

In a nondisplaced fracture, a bone breaks but does not move out of position "Hairline fracture" is a lay term commonly used to describe a subtle nondisplaced fracture. In some cases of nondisplaced fracture, there is very little change visible on X-ray, and in others it is more obvious.

In an incomplete fracture, the fracture goes part way through the bone. An incomplete fracture can be "angulated" or "nonangulated."

If a fracture, whether complete or incomplete, is significantly angulated, there will be a visible deformity. Straightening a displaced, angulated fracture is known as "reduction." More strictly speaking, if a fracture is incomplete but angulated, it is usually easy to straighten by simply bending it back straight again as the splint is applied. If a fracture is complete, displaced, and angulated, reduction can be difficult. The two pieces of bone may be overlapping (overriding), and pulling the extremity back out to length and returning the fracture site to proper alignment can require a lot of force and be very uncomfortable without good anesthesia.

A fracture can also be a "simple fracture," if the bone is broken into two pieces. Simple fractures can be transverse, going straight across the bone, or longitudinal, running lengthwise along the bone. A simple fracture can also be "spiral," though a spiral fracture would usually be simply called spiral. Spiral fractures occur when a twisting force is present as the bone breaks.

If a bone is broken into multiple pieces, it is a "comminuted fracture." In a comminuted fracture, the bone may be fragmented, with multiple pieces, but not necessarily displaced.

An open fracture occurs when the bone protrudes through the skin. An open fracture is sometimes called a "compound fracture." Most frequently, the bone will protrude through the skin at the moment of the trauma, but then be drawn back inside. Usually the injured extremity is deformed, and there is bleeding from the site where the bone came through the skin, often glazed with fat globules from the bone marrow. Open fractures require surgery in the operating room in almost all cases. The surgery for an open fracture must be done right away and is usually scheduled for "zero to four hours" by the orthopedist.

The concern with open fractures is that when the bone broke through the skin, it likely gathered dirt or other foreign material (possibly grinding right into the dirt or on the road) that is now internalized. Without prompt and proper removal, this contamination guarantees a dangerous, deep infection. Serious infection will almost certainly occur if the wound is not opened, explored, and debrided (dirt scraped, scrubbed, or cut away)—as we will discuss in the chapter on wounds.

If a fracture enters a joint space, it is called an "intra-articular fracture." Intra-articular fractures are associated with additional problems, including a high risk of arthritis of the affected joint, and should always be seen by an orthopedist within a week or so of the ER visit.

All of this fracture nomenclature is a bit confusing but just remember: simple vs. comminuted, open versus closed, and displaced versus nondisplaced, and you will do fine.

Fractures in Children

Some pediatric fractures are worth mentioning. In children, "greenstick" fractures are common. This is a bending of the bone with a break in only one side. They may be either displaced or nondisplaced, but there is usually some degree of angulation, though not always enough to demand reduction. A "torus fracture" is another pediatric fracture where a bone is stressed, and a small bump shows on the bone. These are very stable, and generally the child can still use the injured body part. Sometimes they do not even need splinting, though a splint may help with comfort.

Since children who are still growing taller have growth plates, fractures can affect these areas. Growth plates are lines of cartilage (the rubbery part of chicken that is tougher than fat, but softer than bone) through bone where the bone is actively growing. Fractures involving the growth plate are called "Salter" type fractures. They are further broken down into five kinds, each of which has a different appearance and potential effect on the growth of the bone. Knowing which of the five types of fracture your child has is not very important when you see or hear that the fracture affects the growth plate. Ask if growth will be affected, and get an orthopedic referral.

In children, "remodeling" of the bone can help to return a slightly crooked bone to normal shape after an injury. Bones not only become stronger in response to stress, they also change their shape to perform best. Less remodeling of shape occurs in adults, and therefore the fractures must be reduced more exactly in adults.

Reduction Afield?

If you are hiking in rugged country, riding horses, rock climbing, or undertaking some other form of rough activity far from medical help, you may be faced with deciding if a fracture or dislocation needs to be reduced immediately, or whether you should splint the injury and wait until the ED to have it reduced. If there is a change in color or decrease in pulse of the affected extremity, the fracture or dislocation may be putting pressure on an artery, and it should be reduced, or at least straightened, right away before splinting. If there is numbness or decreased ability to move the injured arm or leg, there may be pressure on the nerve, and the displaced fracture or dislocation should once again be reduced right away. Continued pressure on the nerve or artery can cause permanent damage.

Often the best approach to take in the field is to pull the injured arm or leg "back out to length" while applying the splint. This may not result in a complete reduction of the fracture, but will often restore the circulation and nerve function. If the extremity has been without normal blood flow for more than a few minutes, it will usually flush bright red when circulation is first returned.

If you go to an ER with an extremity fracture, what will matter most to you is whether or not it is displaced. If the fracture is displaced, it will need to be straightened or reduced.

If it is a finger or toe fracture, a digital nerve block will often be used. We will discuss the digital nerve block in the "Wounds and Wound Repair" chapter, since it is used even more frequently for finger-laceration repair. After the digit is numb, it will be restored to position.

The commonest dislocated digital fracture of the hand and foot is probably the fifth finger or toe. With the hand, it is often a ball that comes at speed, hitting only the little finger and leaving it in an unnatural looking splayed out position. With the foot, it is usually the fifth (pinkie) toe versus a piece of heavy furniture. The little toe is then pointing outward.

Once the finger or toe is numb, I straighten the broken bone. A common method that works in this scenario is inserting one of my fingers or a pen as a lever between the base of the fifth and fourth fingers, and then squeezing together the fingers that are beyond (distal to) the pen (lever). In this way leverage is applied to the site of the fracture.

If you are a long way from medical help, straightening or relocating a deformed body part may be required and often can be done painlessly if done immediately after the injury occurs. Often there is a period of a few minutes before it really starts hurting.

After reduction the smallest toe or finger is taped to the fourth toe or finger, with a small bit of gauze inserted between. This is known as "buddy taping." The normal toe or finger will help to stabilize the fracture.

One of the most common, painful, and dramatic-looking displaced fractures that needs to be anesthetized and reduced in the ER is a fracture of both bones in the forearm. Having a "second elbow" midway between the wrist and elbow is just no fun! Wrist fractures from falls are also impressive looking and painful. Sometimes these fractures are severely displaced, and great force is required to bring them back to length and normal position.

Anesthesia for Fracture Reduction

There are a number of ways to control the pain as a fracture is reduced in the ER. If the ED is not too busy and there are dedicated nurses available, deep sedation can be used. Be sure the physician discusses the risks of deep sedation with you and offers other options as well.

I was fortunate to learn an excellent technique for "whole arm" anesthesia from my father during medical school, and I have taught the technique to thousands of physicians since that time. This technique is called the "axillary nerve block" (ANB), so named because it is performed in the axilla (armpit).

My father, James Borden, MD, was an orthopedist who specialized in the hand. He performed the vast majority of his surgeries at the San Diego Hand Surgery and Rehabilitation Center and did the anesthesia himself. During his career he did more than nine thousand axillary nerve blocks for presurgical anesthesia. There were no complications beyond the occasional bruise at the injection site, and one case of hand tingling that persisted for three weeks. During the years he was practicing, the same number of cases done under general anesthesia (being "knocked out") would have resulted (statistically speaking) in two deaths attributable to the anesthesia alone and numerous other serious complications requiring a hospital stay. He did not perform regional rather than general anesthesia to save those two lives, though. He did it because it was faster and much cheaper (not having to hire an anesthesiologist and another nurse), and because he was able to talk to the patients during their surgery. I remember hearing him talk to people about fishing spots, stock prices, and a host of other things while I was assisting in the operating room.

The nerves, arteries, and veins that serve the arm all come together on the arm before the arm joins the body. They are surrounded by a covering called a "sheath." With an ANB, a very small needle is used to gently penetrate that sheath where the arm joins the body, and a large amount of local anesthetic, usually lidocaine, is injected into the sheath. The lidocaine then is absorbed into the nerves over a period of five to thirty minutes, numbing the arm from the mid-upper arm to the fingertips. This block provides blessed relief of pain in cases of displaced arm fractures and serious burns. For longer duration, a longer-lasting anesthetic such as Marcaine can be used.

The progression of anesthesia in an axillary nerve block is an interesting study in neurophysiology (how nerves work). Almost immediately after the injection, the pain at rest is gone. The pain and sensory (feeling) nerve fibers are not as thickly insulated (myelinated) as the motor (movement) fibers. The arm can still move normally initially, and in fact soon can move much better than before the nerve block, since there is no pain. The triceps muscle is almost always the first to lose its strength. After the anesthetic is fully absorbed, much of the strength of movement goes away, as well. I warn patients with forearm fractures not to try to scratch their faces. Since the excruciating pain in the arm is gone, patients are tempted to use the arm normally, but since they are lying on their back, "thump"—they accidentally hit their nose with the numb hand, rather than scratching it!

The ANB is the best method of anesthesia if a displaced forearm fracture needs to be straightened. Though more and more emergency physicians are using the ANB, some are not familiar with the technique. If your emergency physician is not familiar with the procedure, and you are in a large hospital, an anesthesiologist can be called down, and they are generally able to perform the procedure. Another option in smaller hospitals is to have your physician visit the medical section of my personal website, www.windroseenterprises.com, where he or she can learn the technique. The technique taught on my website is safe, highly effective, and very simple. The technique is even easier with ultrasound guidance.

After the arm is good and numb, the fracture is reduced. This is sometimes as easy as straightening the arm, but if the fracture is complete, it is often much more difficult. To reduce a fracture, the arm must be pulled back out to length and the bone ends set atop one another again. I usually use "finger traps" hung from an IV pole to help. Finger traps are those things you stick your finger into and when you try to pull your finger out, they tighten, squeezing the finger. The weight of the numb arm helps the arm return to normal length and maintain the reduction after it is back in place. The arm, looking much better now, is splinted to maintain position. A post-reduction X-ray is then usually taken to show that the reduction is satisfactory.

An ankle nerve block is great for the reduction of an ankle fracture, and there is nothing better for the pain of a femur fracture than a femoral nerve block. Not only is the pain relieved, but the painful spasm of the strong quadriceps muscles is eliminated.

Will I get a Splint, or a Cast?

Extremity fractures that occurred shortly before arrival to the ED will be splinted, rather than casted. A splint only partially encircles the extremity with hard material, so if further swelling occurs, the splint can loosen, and circulation will continue. After the swelling has decreased, usually at the end of the first week, the splint can be replaced with a cast. The cast provides better support and protection. If the cast were placed while the arm was swollen, even if the swelling had reached maximum, a different problem would occur. The cast would need to be replaced in a week anyway, because when the swelling went down, it would be too loose to support the arm properly.

Spinal Fractures

Spinal fractures are potentially very serious, and a careful neurological exam is needed. Expect the news that you have a spine fracture to come with quite a bit of an explanation and possibly more testing to determine the extent and stability of the fracture. A minor, stable spinal fracture may need no additional care beyond pain medication. A serious fracture may require a "halo," which is a metal ring around the head, secured with screws to the skull and anchored with metal rods to a rigid vest. They look rather uncomfortable, to say the least. Surgical repair may also be needed for serious fractures.

Almost all mammals, including humans, have seven neck (cervical) vertebrae. Even the giraffe only has seven!

Chapter 21 Fractures and Dislocations

Some cervical spine fractures cause death because, when associated with complete spinal cord injury, they cause paralysis of the entire body. This paralysis includes the diaphragm and chest wall, so breathing stops. Fractures between the third and seventh cervical vertebrae allow continued breathing, but can severely decrease hand and arm function.

The nerves that power the arms come from the neck and the first level of the thorax, so neck fractures can affect the arms, whereas fractures of the mid and lower thoracic region do not. When you see paraplegics pushing the wheels of their wheelchair with their hands, you can be sure, if they are doing a good, strong job, that their injury is below the neck. If they have a stable and strong chest, back, and abdomen, which is required to do a very good job, as in wheelchair races, you can be sure their injury is to the lowest thoracic level or lumbar level.

As can be inferred from above, thoracic spinal injuries affect the muscles of the chest wall, back, and abdominal wall. A complete thoracic injury will, of course, block conduction of the nerves to the legs, as well. There are twelve thoracic vertebrae, which have the twelve ribs attached to them.

Fractures of the lumbar spine and upper sacrum affect the legs. Sexual function is also affected by injuries to this region. There are five lumbar vertebrae in the low back. The sciatic nerve, which we discussed in the "Back Pain" chapter, comes from the low lumbar and upper sacral spine.

In the elderly, "spinal compression fractures" are common. These certainly look painful on X-rays, but the pain experienced by the patient can vary from mild to severe. This fracture is a vertical collapse of the vertebral body and usually does not cause nerve problems. This vertical collapse is one of the reasons why people get shorter as they get older. The thick cartilage pads between the spinal bones (intervertebral discs) also become thinner, causing a further loss of height. Compression fractures are often in the thoracic spine and thus do not usually cause serious nerve symptoms. They can cause shooting pains and other sensations that wrap around the thorax or abdomen along the paths of the involved nerves.

Dislocations

Dislocations are a relatively common problem. When we discussed ligaments in the "Extremity Pain after Trauma" chapter, I explained that they hold the joints in position. If all of the muscle and other overlying tissue were removed from the body, the skeleton would look like the ones that hung in the back of our laboratory at medical school; the ligaments would be holding the bones together in place.

Ligaments allow the normal range of motion of a joint, but to exceed that normal range, a ligament needs to "give." Ligaments can be stretched a bit and loosened slightly with repeated stress, but it is uncomfortable and difficult. Ligaments are not made to be loosened. When a ligament is partially torn, the joint is sometimes less stable, and this instability can result in pain and arthritis. Stretching exercises normally increase muscle and tendon length and muscle range of motion. Flexibility gains come mainly from the changes to muscle and tendons, not from changes to ligaments.

When a joint is dislocated, a ligament or ligaments must have been either disrupted completely or injured and pushed aside to allow the bone to move out of position. If a joint has been dislocated before, and the ligaments have not healed completely, it can dislocate again more easily.

Patients often think that after a dislocation is "popped back in," all the trouble is over, but that is not usually the case. The ligaments are still injured and will need to either heal, or if completely disrupted, be repaired by an orthopedist.

Chapter 21 Fractures and Dislocations

Dislocations are painful, especially until they are "reduced," and there is usually an obvious deformity. When you see a dislocation on the athletic field or during recreational activities, it will often be hard to be sure it is not a "fracture-dislocation." Whether or not there is a fracture, if there is impaired circulation or nerve function, you will still need to reduce the injury, or see that it is done promptly, as we discussed above.

Reducing a Shoulder Dislocation

Shoulder dislocations are common and tend to be recurrent. People who have recurrent shoulder dislocations can learn to "put their shoulder back in" by themselves. Learning self-reduction is a good idea if a person does not plan to have an orthopedic repair to increase stability.

To determine whether a person's shoulder is dislocated, feel along the clavicle until you reach the hard bone on top of the shoulder known as the acromion. The clavicle (collar bone) connects into the acromion, which is the top part of the scapula (shoulder blade). Sometimes a broken clavicle will imitate a dislocated shoulder. If the clavicle is crooked, swollen, or very tender, you may have found the problem. When you get to the acromion, there should be the same shape and connection to the clavicle as is present on the person's other side. Feel the other side for a reference.

Continuing outward, you will next feel the deltoid muscle. When it is in position, the head of the humerus, which is the big bone in the upper arm, "fills out" the deltoid muscle, making the shoulders look wider. In a shoulder dislocation, the humeral head is no longer under the deltoid muscle, so it collapses inward, leaving a depression under the acromion. If you feel around, you can locate the displaced humerus, which is usually moved toward the front of the shoulder and padded by the front of the deltoid muscle. Compared to the other shoulder, the deltoid muscle will feel sunken and collapsed on the dislocated side.

If you need to reduce a dislocated shoulder, there are several methods to try. Since you will not have sedation, the major problem to overcome is the muscular tension caused by pain and apprehension. If the person is resisting your attempts, reducing the shoulder is much harder. This resistance is overcome by proceeding slowly. Keeping yourself in the position of greatest strength and leverage allows you to "wear out" the person's muscles slowly as he or she relaxes, and the shoulder should ease, or "pop," back in place.

The first technique I usually try is the "external rotation technique." This is also known as Kocher's method. This can be harder in the field, unless you have a bed or gurney. It can be done on a table or the tailgate of a pickup if needed. Have the person lie on his/her back with the dislocated arm on the edge of an elevated, flat surface. Keep the arm bent ninety degrees at the elbow throughout. Bring the elbow in to the person's side and keep it there with one hand. With the other hand, turn the hand and forearm outward (external rotation). Go very slowly. It will likely take at least several minutes to get the hand to or below the level of the bed. If the shoulder has not reduced when the hand is below the level of the bed, keep it there while the muscles relax. The shoulder will usually pop in within a few minutes. Try rubbing the front of the shoulder a bit. You will feel the humeral head well in this position.

If the external rotation technique does not work, the next one to try in the field is the "Eskimo technique," or a variation thereof. The patient lies on the uninjured side, and two people lift straight upward, by the hand and wrist, on the injured arm. When the patient is able to relax, or when his/her arm tires, the shoulder will relocate. A single person may have trouble with this method.

Another variation is to sit at the patient's side (the patient is on his/her back) facing the axilla on the injured side. Padding the axilla (armpit) with a towel to prevent discomfort, put one of your feet in the person's armpit, and grasp the wrist with your hands. Encourage the person to relax, and then lean back, pulling downward on the arm. You are now seated in a rowing position and have good leverage. The shoulder should reduce with a "pop" or "clunk" as the patient relaxes.

After reduction, an X-ray is done in the ER to confirm position and look for possible fractures. In the field or at home, you will need to rely on the fact that the deltoid is no longer collapsed/sunken and that the patient can now move the arm once again. Great pain relief is immediate after the shoulder is reduced, as well. A sling or shoulder immobilizer is then applied.

Sometimes sedation is needed in the ER to reduce a dislocation, and some pain medication is often needed afterward if the dislocation was traumatic, rather than recurrent.

Another shoulder injury that occurs commonly is an "acromio-clavicular dislocation," also known as a "shoulder separation." A shoulder separation will be visible externally, since the end of the clavicle farthest from the neck (distal clavicle) will be sticking up above the level of the acromion. The connection between the clavicle and acromion is not important for function, and a sling is usually the only treatment. This joint (the acromioclavicular, or AC, joint) can be reduced easily by lifting up on the arm, but there is no tendency for it to stay in position, and as soon as you release the arm, it will dislo-cate again. In an AC separation, unlike with shoulder dislocation, the deltoid muscle will not be sunken.

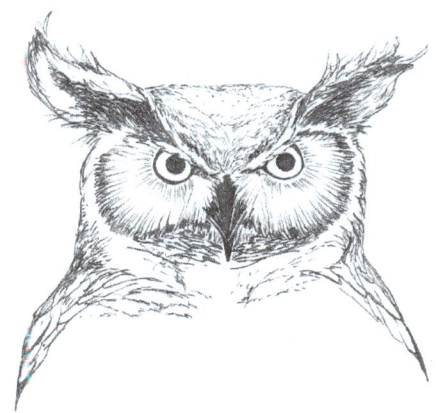

Chapter 22
Gastrointestinal Bleeding

I will prescribe regimens for the good of my patients according to
my ability and my judgment and never do harm to anyone.

—from a translation of the original Hippocratic Oath, circa 400 BC

Minor bleeding with the passage of hard stool is not uncommon, since abrasions around the rectum or hemorrhoids can bleed a little. More than a small amount of blood from the rectum, though, brings a lot of people to the ER.

Lots of bright red blood is clearly a serious problem, but sometimes rectal bleeding can be subtle. If the bowel movements are brown, but anemia is present, testing the stool for "occult" blood is done with testing cards and developer. If a large amount of blood is lost from a higher level, such as the stomach, but then not vomited, it will darken as it moves down the intestinal tract, eventually becoming black. "Dark tarry stool" is a description your doctor will use. Melena is the medical word for black stool that contains "digested" blood. Black stools can also result from iron pills and Pepto Bismol, so a black stool may need to be tested for occult blood.

If a source of bleeding above the rectum is suspected, your doctor may recommend endoscopy, which is "taking a look up there" or "down there" with a long flexible tool called an endoscope. In upper endoscopy, the endoscope is passed through the mouth to look at the esophagus, stomach, and duodenum. In lower endoscopy, the endoscope is passed through the anus to visualize the rectum and large intestine. There is an area of small bowel that cannot be visualized from either above or below, but luckily that area is relatively trouble free. Most of the problems happen toward the two ends.

Some problems can be visualized by doing barium studies of the bowel. Barium is a dense liquid that blocks X-ray transmission and thus shows up as white on an X-ray. Bones also show up as white, but barium is even denser and therefore even whiter than bone on the X-ray. An X-ray taken immediately after swallowing barium will outline the esophagus and, about ten to twenty seconds later, the stomach.

Occasionally I will use a "barium swallow" to look for an esophageal foreign body or obstruction. Once I treated a man who had swallowed something he would not mention, but which he felt was stuck in his chest. He pointed at his sternum. He seemed a bit restless and preoccupied and was pacing at his bedside, so we gave him some medication to relax him while I ordered a swallow study and an abdominal series (see the "X-Ray and Radiology" chapter). The abdominal series came back first, and it was very strange. It showed a bunch of variably seen, vague objects that were hard to identify. Eighteen were clearly seen, and several were, upon more detailed study, small doll heads! A partially obstructing object was in the esophagus, and that one had to be removed by our gastroenterologist. It was indeed, a blonde Barbie doll head! I admitted the patient to the hospital, since there was a chance that the heads would cause obstruction at the next tight spot—the junction of the small and large bowel. I couldn't resist asking why, and to this he replied that it "was the right thing to do." He later told one of my residents, "It was an accident." He would need another specialty to consult during his time in the hospital, of course!

Upper endoscopy is useful for inspection of the throat, esophagus, stomach, duodenum, and a bit of intestine. Upper endoscopy can also help you if you accidentally swallow nineteen Barbie doll heads and are unfortunate enough to have the long, blond hair of the last one block your esophagus! Upper endoscopy is also indicated when injury of or bleeding from the stomach and/or esophagus is suspected.

Vomiting of blood can occur after repeated emesis from food poisoning or gastroenteritis (stomach flu). Typically there is a small amount of blood, which may appear darkened or look like coffee grounds. In this instance, the vomit initially is blood free, but the repeated vomiting can cause a small tear, known as a "Mallory Weiss tear." This is not generally a serious problem. Medication to stop the vomiting should be given, and acid-blocking medications may also help.

An ulcer of the stomach or esophagus can cause pain and bleeding, and often the bleeding is enough to be frightening. In this case, seek medical attention promptly.

Alcohol abuse and liver disease can cause serious bleeding complications. Alcohol alone can cause painful stomach injury known as gastritis. If the liver is scarred (cirrhosis), and the blood flow to it is slowed, pressure can build in the big thin-walled veins of the esophagus, which are known as "esophageal varices." If these bleed, the blood loss can be massive and life threatening. Bleeding of this sort is known as "variceal bleeding" and tends to be recurrent and problematic in patients with liver disease.

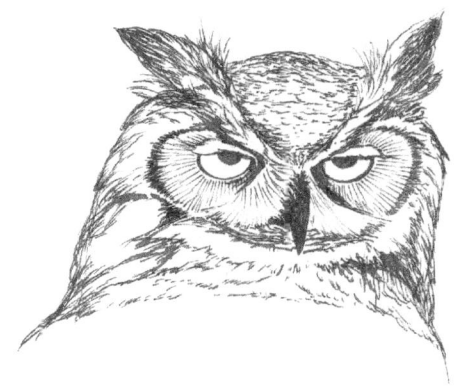

Chapter 23
Headache

My son complains about headaches. I tell him all the time, when you get out of bed, it's feet first!

—Henny Youngman

If the headache can be reproduced or changed with palpation of the muscles and nerves of the posterior neck, it can be relieved with a properly placed injection of local anesthetic.

—BoThomas Brofeldt MD, professor UC Davis Medical Center

The first thing your doctor in the ER will want to determine when you go there with a headache is: is this a serious, life-threatening headache.

or is it just another headache? Many people have headaches every day. Sometimes these are mild and can either be ignored or treated with Tylenol/ibuprofen, but sometimes they are more severe and may require ongoing treatment. There are a handful of things that cause a potentially damaging headache, and we will cover these in detail.

Some things will cause anyone to have a headache. These include neck-muscle tightness and poor neck posture, bright lights and other causes of eye strain, chemical smells, inhalation of carbon monoxide (exhaust fumes/smoke), caffeine withdrawal, and dehydration. There are many others, which vary from individual to individual. Certainly most of these headaches can be treated with Tylenol or ibuprofen, but relieving/removing the cause makes more sense. Inhalation of smoke/fumes in small amounts causes a headache, but a bit more can be fatal, so in that case the headache is a warning and should certainly be heeded.

Muscle Tension Headache

Muscle-tension headaches are commonly seen in the ER and are often mislabeled as "migraines." During my residency training, I worked with an emergency physician named Dr. Bo Thomas Brofeldt. Dr. Brofeldt pioneered and researched a technique of local anesthetic injection of the nerves that come up on either side of the occipital area where the neck meets the head. Those nerves supply sensation to the scalp, and muscle spasm can compress and irritate them, causing pain in the head. The pain is felt within the head, but injection of the nerves causes instant relief of pain in a very high percentage of patients, many of whom had been treated for migraines for many years. I saw many patients hugging Dr. Brofeldt after his injections and heard a number of patients say, "I now (that it is gone) realize that I have been living with that headache for as long as I can remember."

Muscle-tension headaches usually improve to at least some extent when the patient lies down, with the neck in a comfortable neutral position. Ibuprofen or Tylenol also helps, though relief is often not usually complete. Improving posture can help. If you spend a lot of time on the computer, raise the monitor so your neck is in a more neutral position. If your physician does posterior occipital injections—and Dr. Brofeldt's technique is widely known and practiced—an injection of long-lasting local anesthetic can work miracles. The problem will likely return, though, so causes should be considered.

Migraine

Migraine headaches are less clear in their cause, but are felt to occur as a result of changes in blood flow within the brain. Our neurology professor gave us the classic description of a migraine: "Shh, Mommy's got a sick headache." This sentence includes the young female predominance, the sound (and light) sensitivity, and the vomiting. Migraines are common in youngish females, but certainly occur in others as well.

There are many specific treatments for migraine, and sometimes pain and nausea medication is also needed. If the nausea and vomiting has been severe or of long duration, rehydration may be needed.

If a person has recurrent migraines, or recurrent severe headaches of any type, having a personal physician or neurologist is a good idea. Frequent visits to the ER for headache will result in poor care, and I have witnessed several very bad outcomes, including addiction and overdose, as a result. Many ERs will not give narcotics for recurrent headache, and most have a policy for the treatment of chronic pain.

Is the Headache an Emergency?

Dangerous causes of headache that must be recognized and treated include: spontaneous bleeding in the brain, brain infection, brain tumor, and arteritis. We will discuss each of these in turn.

Medical Wisdom

Spontaneous bleeding in the brain takes several forms. The form we worry about with sudden onset of severe headache is called subarachnoid hemorrhage (SAH). This bleeding is caused by an arterial rupture at a weak spot, usually near the base of the brain. The weak spot is considered to be congenital (present at birth) in most cases. The blood goes into the cerebrospinal fluid, causing irritation of the sensitive linings that surround the brain.

The pain of a subarachnoid hemorrhage is typically sudden in onset, severe, and unlike normal headaches. Doctors are taught to think of this headache when someone says: (1) "This is the worst headache I have ever had," and (2) "This is unlike any headache I have had before." A CT scan (described in the "X-Ray and Radiology" chapter) can help to identify this sort of headache, and a CT is most accurate if done within the first few hours. Sampling the spinal fluid with a lumbar puncture is a more definitive test, and we are taught to perform a lumbar puncture if the CT is normal but a subarachnoid hemorrhage is still suspected.

If identified, a SAH can be treated surgically. If not identified in time, death may result. A friend of my wife's was at home with her husband when he suddenly grabbed his head in pain, saying he had a bad headache and needed to lie down. He was in his early forties and had never complained of headaches, so she was concerned. He also became sweaty, was breathing hard, and vomited once into the sink. He made it to the couch, but lying down didn't help. She offered to call the doctor or an ambulance, but he said he would be OK. When she came back to check on him a few minutes later, he wasn't breathing! She called the ambulance and started CPR, but he was declared dead at the scene.

Though there are occasions when a subarachnoid hemorrhage can cause less dramatic symptoms, most cases I have seen were very serious, and the person was in obvious distress. Vomiting is common, as are changes in blood pressure, heart rate, and breathing.

Chapter 23 Headache

Hemorrhagic (bleeding in the brain) stroke accounts for about 10 percent of all strokes. A bleeding stroke can cause a severe headache or no headache at all, depending on the location in the brain. The subarachnoid hemorrhage we discussed above is usually painful, since it occurs in the vessels near the brain and contacts the sensitive membranes (meninges) that surround the brain. The white and grey matter of the brain itself is not sensitive to pain. If a bleed occurs within the brain tissue itself, it may be painless.

Increases in pressure can cause pain, if the bleeding is substantial. Increased pressure within the skull is the major problem when there is bleeding within the brain. The skull is a closed compartment, and pressure can only escape through the entrance of the spinal cord, at its base. Increased spinal fluid pressure can move into the spinal cord initially, but then severe problems occur. Pressure on the brain stem from the brain trying to "squeeze through" the base of the skull as pressure increases causes the pupils to change. The nerves that control the pupils (cranial nerves) are located in the brain stem, and pressure on them stops their function. Changes in the pupils is a late sign of brain bleeding, though, since the source of consciousness is also located in the brain stem, and the person will lose consciousness before the pupils change.

When a patient arrives in the ER with a stroke, a CT is done promptly to differentiate between a bleeding stroke and a clotting (ischemic—not enough blood flow) stroke. If there is bleeding, the neurosurgeon is called. We will discuss the clotting/ischemic stroke in the "Weakness" chapter.

Brain infection (meningitis and encephalitis) causes a severe headache. A high and persistent fever is usually present, and the patient feels "sick." Bacterial meningitis is very serious and needs to be identified and treated with antibiotics as early as possible. A lumbar puncture (spinal tap) is needed to identify meningitis.

It is safe to say that a bad cold (viral infection) with a bad head-ache causes some degree of "meningitis" because a viral infection pretty much inflames the whole body, head included. The lumbar puncture in this case will show some mild signs of inflammation, but the types of cells, the much milder degree of inflammation, and the lack of visible bacteria makes it possible to reassure the patient in these cases.

Temporal arteritis is an inflammation of the artery in the temple. This causes pain in the temple and also a headache of varying type and severity. Temporal arteritis is a serious problem and can lead to blindness if not treated. The artery in the temple is tender to touch and swollen to some extent. Temporal arteritis is commonest in mid to late life. If you have a headache that is new to you, and there is tenderness, be sure to mention it to your doctor.

Severe, sudden, and sharp pains can occur in the face and head. There are a number of causes of sharp, knifelike pain, and "neural-gia" is the word used to describe that sort of pain. There are some specific treatments for neuralgia, so if you or someone you know suffers from sharp, stabbing, recurrent facial or head pain, it is worth seeing a physician.

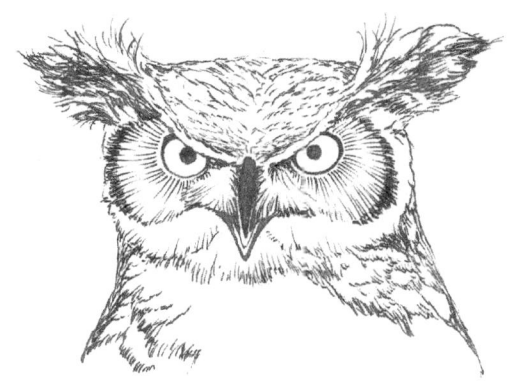

Chapter 24
Head Injury

One should not bring sympathy to a sick man. It is always kindly meant, and of course it has to be taken—but it isn't much of an improvement on castor oil. One who has a sick man's true interest at heart will forbear spoken sympathy, and bring him surreptitious soup and fried oysters and other trifles that the doctor has tabooed.

—Mark Twain

Head injury can certainly cause a headache, but a "bump on the head" should cause the same sort of pain as a "bump on the shoulder." A serious impact (of the sort that might cause you to consider a trip to the ER) is a different matter. Not only will the site of impact be tender and painful, but the pain might be deeper, more severe, and can be accompanied by disturbing symptoms such as memory loss, weakness, numbness, and possibly recurrent vomiting.

So how do you decide when head injury merits a trip to the ER? Good reasons to see a physician promptly include a serious impact causing loss of consciousness or decrease in alertness, significant swelling, bleeding/laceration, persistent vomiting, or severe head pain. A common sign of serious head injury is repetitive questioning. It is often almost comical when a seemingly alert patient asks the same question dozens of times, despite receiving an answer each time. Well-meaning friends will at first answer the question more fully and in greater and greater detail, with the patient acknowledging them each time thankfully, but eventually even they give up!

In the case of a child, any noticeable alteration in behavior after a head injury is reason to suspect a problem. A child should cry immediately at the time of injury, but after a few minutes should be consolable. Though a single episode of vomiting often occurs after even a minor head injury, persistent vomiting should prompt a call to the doctor or a trip to the ER.

The head is different from most other body parts because the skull forms a closed compartment. When bleeding occurs within the skull, there is an increase in pressure. If the bleeding connects to the cerebrospinal fluid, which surrounds the brain and spinal cord, the pressure can be evenly distributed. If the bleeding does not connect to the cerebrospinal fluid, the pressure can build in the head, forcing the soft and sensitive lower-brain structures out through the place where the spinal cord enters the skull. We discussed this briefly in the preceding chapter. This problem is obviously very serious, and is called "herniation."

When the brain begins to be forced out of the skull, pressure is felt by some nerves, one of which controls the pupil. Unequal pupils are something people always look for in head injury, but unequal pupils are a late sign that arises after, or at the same time as, consciousness is lost. If someone with unequal pupils is talking to you, they probably either rubbed a medicine in the eye that caused the pupil to dilate, were born with unequal pupils, or have an injury of that eye. Twice in the last year, I have treated patients who complained of an unequal pupil. Both of them had recently applied stick-on patches to prevent seasickness. Ah…to live near the sea!

Head Injuries from the Outside In

Starting from the outside, the scalp is frequently subject to contusion and laceration. Lacerations to the scalp are not as important cosmetically (unless a person is or "plans to" go bald!) as those of the face, and they are often contaminated, both by hair and by other material, such as dirt. As with all lacerations, these wounds should be thoroughly cleansed.

One of the commonest medically related infections occurs when a small scalp laceration is sutured. If the laceration is less than one centimeter long, it is almost certainly deeper than it is long and therefore should be considered a puncture wound. We discussed puncture wounds and their treatment in the "Bites and Stings" chapter, but to repeat, they should never be closed by suturing. There is usually a collection of blood (hematoma) beneath the small scalp laceration, and a collection of blood is especially prone to infection when seeded with bacteria from a puncture.

The best time to ensure there is no skull fracture is before the wound is repaired. The physician should explore the wound both visually and manually. Many skull fractures (indicating the previously unsuspected possibility of brain injury) are found during wound exploration. A skull fracture is very obvious when felt with a gloved finger through an open wound.

Facial wounds sometimes require multiple-layer closure to ensure that the facial muscles are repaired and facial expression is preserved. With scalp wounds, muscle repair is less important. A multiple-layer closure (burying deep stitches) contributes to the chance of infection by adding foreign material to the wound. Even though the suture is sterile, the wound is not, and bleeding will accumulate around the sutures, serving as a potential starting place of infection.

There are a number of ways to repair a scalp wound besides the conventional sutures (stitches). Staples are considered acceptable on the scalp, and they have the advantage of being less reactive and quicker to place than sutures. The main disadvantage of staples arises at the time of removal. A special medical staple remover is needed, whereas sutures can be removed at home with a scissor and tweezers in most cases.

After numbing and thorough cleansing/exploration, a scalp wound that is not too deep can often be closed by a technique called "hair tying," which is self-explanatory. A technique I use on occasion when a scalp wound is not too deep is to cross two small bunches of hair over the cleansed wound, adjusting directions until the wound looks right, and then apply a small bit of wound glue to the wound edge and crossed hairs. For shallow scalp wounds, this works well. We will discuss the specific considerations of wound care again in the "Wounds and Wound Repair" chapter.

Scalp lacerations tend to bleed a lot. Applying firm, direct pressure will work to stop it, as in most cases of bleeding. Also it is good to know that the blood supply to the scalp comes up from the face and neck, rather than from within the head, and thus can be stopped with a tight headband. Bleeding can be controlled somewhat by using a local anesthetic that contains epinephrine (adrenaline), which is a vasoconstrictor (makes vessels tighten up). Stapling and "figure-eight sutures" will also sometimes be used to stop bleeding, and the staples or tight suture later removed for final repair after other, more pressing injuries have been stabilized.

The skull bone or "calvarium" is the next level beneath the scalp. Skull fractures are important to discover. A blow to the head that is hard enough to cause a skull fracture will usually (though not always) result in a loss of consciousness. The presence of a skull fracture increases the risk of brain injury and bleeding within and around the brain.

Twenty years ago, I often looked for skull fractures with "plain films" (simple, unidirectional X-rays), but CT (computed tomography) is now the commonest test. CT (sometimes referred to as a brain scan or "cat" scan) is also useful for finding bleeding in the head and brain injury. The down side of CT is the high radiation dose. A head CT is equal in radiation to about 250 standard X-rays and therefore should only be done if needed. We will discuss the various X-ray tests in the "X-Ray and Radiology" chapter.

There are four different types of bleeding within the skull, and we will start from the outermost layer. The first type of bleeding is referred to as "epidural" bleeding. The brain is surrounded by a fairly tough, fibrous layer of tissue that feels like thin, wet canvas. If a skull fracture or serious blow causes the arteries that run along this outer layer to bleed, a bleed of arterial (highest) pressure can accumulate between the brain and the skull. This pressure can push on the brain, deforming it and causing the deadly problem of herniation we discussed above.

Epidural bleeds are often seen in young patients, and the classic story describes a "lucid interval" after an initial loss of consciousness. The initial impact causes the loss of brain conduction and loss of consciousness, but then the person wakes up. The bleeding has begun, and as pressure builds, the brain is displaced, resulting in the tendency of the brain to be pushed out of the skull. There is only one potential exit for the pressure, and that is through the base of the skull, where the spinal cord enters. This movement results in pressure on the lower brain (brain stem), and consciousness is lost again. Pupils will then be unequal or nonreactive, and unless pressure is quickly relieved, death will follow.

This series of events (herniation, loss of consciousness, death) only occurs in "closed-head injury." A skull fracture and open scalp laceration can prevent this problem by allowing the blood to exit the skull, rather than building up within the skull. The treatment is the same: drilling through the skull into the area of blood collection (hematoma) to allow drainage and relieve pressure on the brain. This procedure is called "burr-hole placement."

A difficult situation occurs when an epidural hematoma is recognized in a small hospital that has no neurosurgeon. Many emergency physicians are trained in burr-hole placement, but some are not, as this is not a procedure we do regularly. If the patient is still lucid when the epidural bleed is found, there is a strong argument for immediate transport to a facility with a neurosurgeon. If the patient loses consciousness, however, transport of more than a few minutes will not be fast enough, and the patient will die.

I took a number of these very difficult calls while at the university, since we had the neurosurgical team, and would receive these patients by helicopter. Once I received a frantic call from a family-medicine-trained physician working in an ER more than an hour from our facility. He had received a fourteen-year-old boy who had hit his head at a skate park two hours earlier. Initially the boy was talking and complained of headache. He had lost consciousness for several minutes at the time of the accident, but then "didn't feel right" and called home for a ride. CT scan showed a fairly large left-sided epidural hematoma. Minutes after the CT, the boy began vomiting uncontrollably and lost consciousness. One pupil was dilated and unresponsive to light. The physician was asking me to accept the patient in transfer.

An hour is too long in this case, and I advised him that drainage of the epidural hematoma was needed immediately and that the patient would not recover if transferred. He had called the general surgeon on call, and his arrival was expected in fifteen minutes. There was a burr-hole kit in the ER. The physician said he was "not comfortable doing the procedure." To this I replied something along the lines of, "It will be better for you to drill a handful of holes with the Makita in your garage than do nothing."

While on speaker phone, I talked him through the procedure. The anesthesiologist was present, managing the ventilator, and he had seen several burr holes done. I could hear him voicing encouragement and then helping as well. The correct side was confirmed by reviewing the CT, the area shaved (over the ear and a bit forward), lidocaine with epinephrine quickly injected, and an incision made through the scalp to the skull. Meanwhile, the drill was assembled by a mechanically capable nurse. The first hole (about a half-inch in diameter) showed dark blood clot, which oozed and then, when suctioned, bled freely.

Within a minute, the patient's eye exam normalized! The pressure had been removed from the brain, and the patient was safe for transport. I could hear the enthusiastic relief of the whole team over the speakerphone. The patient was transported uneventfully and recovered fully, leaving our hospital in less than a week.

Less than a week later, a similar case occurred, but this time the outcome was not favorable. The patient was an eleven-year-old girl who was thrown from a horse, without a helmet, hitting her head on a "pile of rocks, along a fence line." Her sister "couldn't wake her up" at first, but then she woke up and managed to get back on the horse and ride home. She had a small laceration with mild bleeding above her right ear. Her mother brought her to the small ER "for stitches."

Medical Wisdom

In the waiting room, she began to have recurrent vomiting, and after emptying her stomach, continued to dry heave. She complained of a headache. When I received the call from the family doctor who was covering the ER, she was much worse. She lost consciousness shortly after being brought back to her ER bed, and a breathing tube was placed. One of her pupils was "blown" (very large) and unreactive to light. Her CT showed an epidural bleed, with a shift of the right side of the brain toward the left. The helicopter had been called.

I advised the transferring doctor that he or his surgeon needed to relieve the pressure by draining the epidural bleed with a burr hole. He was not trained in emergency medicine and had no experience with burr holes. There was no surgeon available. The medical director of the emergency department was a trained emergency physician that I knew, and had trained, personally. He lived near the hospital and often would have been able to respond from home during such a crisis, but he was not on call, and could not be reached. Increasing the ventilator rate and giving mannitol (two steps that can decrease intracranial pressure a bit) had no effect. I could not persuade the physician to consider the procedure, and certainly "to first do no harm" is an argument that can be used by a reluctant physician in this situation. I advised him that without prompt drainage, her chance of recovery after nearly an hour in transit was very poor. I notified the neurosurgery team, and she went straight to the operating room on arrival at the trauma center. Despite efficient treatment, she did not recover and was declared brain dead in our ICU two days later.

Both of these cases demonstrate the classic "lucid interval" after an initial loss of consciousness. The first six hours is the crucial period with an epidural bleed. If a CT scan is not available and a serious head injury suspected, the patient must be observed closely for at least that long.

Chapter 24 Head Injury

Continuing deeper into the brain, the "subdural hemorrhage" is next. Subdural hemorrhage is a venous type of bleed, rather than arterial, as in the epidural we discussed above, and is thus lower in pressure. The bleeding occurs from the veins beneath the tough dural (outermost) membrane. These veins can become stretched in older age and are also delicate in infants. Subdural bleeding can be more rapidly forming, or slow and insidious. Pressure increase is not as much of a problem as with the arterial bleeds.

Subdural bleeding usually occurs in older patients, and the nursery rhyme about the "old man" describes a subdural: "He bumped his head, went to bed, and couldn't get up in the morning." A seemingly minor head injury can result in this type of bleeding, especially in patients who are taking blood thinners or have blood-clotting problems. Suspect this sort of bleeding if an older person falls or otherwise suffers a head injury and then anytime within a month afterward begins to suffer loss of balance, difficulty with speech, lethargy, persistent nausea and vomiting, or other neurologic change. Treatment can be lifesaving, and a CT scan is diagnostic.

Bleeding within the brain tissue is referred to as "intraparenchymal hemorrhage." This is also called a hemorrhagic stroke (when it occurs without trauma) or "hemorrhagic cerebrovascular accident" (CVA). About 10 percent of strokes are caused by bleeding. Stroke symptoms (weakness of one side, speech difficulty, numbness, paralysis) with headache and blood pressure/heart-rate changes are often seen. In these cases, we call the neurosurgeon, rather than the neurologist, as sometimes surgery is needed.

We discussed the spontaneous bleed from an artery within the brain/at the base of the brain in the "Headache" chapter, as that type of bleeding typically causes a severe headache. Sometimes these other types of bleeding don't cause as much pain, and sometimes they cause no pain, so they should still be suspected if neurologic changes occur.

At this time we use CT scans to look for brain bleeding (injury), but a CT is not as sensitive as an MRI and certainly not as sensitive as tests we will have in the future. An intern of mine once accidentally ordered an MRI, rather than a CT, on a patient who had fallen. The MRI showed a small amount of bleeding, so we called neurosurgery for an opinion. The neurosurgeon didn't know what to do and asked that we order a CT. The CT was completely normal, with no bleeding seen! The neurosurgeon said we should base our treatment decisions on the CT, rather than the MRI, and thus no treatment was indicated. The CT, when done for head injury, is sensitive enough to detect bleeding if there is enough bleeding to need treatment. As you can see, even though the CT is normal, there may still be some brain injury and therefore some symptoms.

Full recovery should be expected if the CT is normal or not needed, even though there may be some symptoms. Transient symptoms after concussion can include dizziness, memory loss, headache, and irritability. Currently there is an emphasis on preventing recurrent concussion. If in doubt, call your doctor. If symptoms of head injury are serious, call 911.

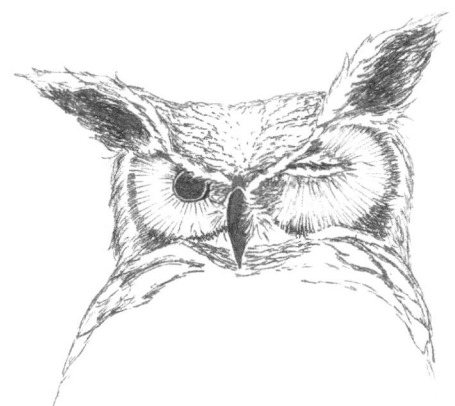

Chapter 25
Hernias

One good thing about music, when it hits—you feel no pain.

—Bob Marley

A hernia occurs when an organ or body part bulges out of the body cavity in which it normally is found. The commonest hernias visible externally are seen in the abdominal wall and inguinal area. Hernias can be annoying or life threatening, and often some of both.

Hernias are associated with weak spots, and the weak spot can be torn/stretched with heavy lifting while tightening the abdomen and closing off the airway (Valsalva maneuver). This raising of the intra-abdominal pressure causes stress on the abdominal wall, and if there is a weak area, pain and herniation at that spot can occur. After a time, the pain goes away. The defect in the abdominal wall heals somewhat, and the hernia can then bulge without pain.

Many children (and puppies) are born with small hernias at the umbilicus. These umbilical hernias will often heal by themselves, but if they do not do so by the time a child is five years old (human years, not dog years!) or if they cause problems, a surgical repair may be needed.

Abdominal-wall hernias can occur spontaneously or via a weak spot in a surgical repair. If abdominal contents bulge from within the abdomen, they should return to the abdomen when pushed. This is called "reduction" of the hernia. Some people live with hernias for many years rather than have surgery, and a device called a "truss" can be used to hold the hernia contents within the abdomen. An inguinal hernia, which is commoner in men, bulges into the scrotum.

When a Hernia "Goes to Jail"

If a hernia that normally goes in and out (bulges and can be reduced/ reduces) suddenly "gets stuck while bulging," the problem can be serious. This occurrence is called "incarceration." When the hernia content becomes incarcerated, the venous (low-pressure) blood vessels can be partially blocked off. Since the arterial (high-pressure) flow to the hernia contents continues, the contents will swell, causing the veins to be further obstructed.

When the veins are completely obstructed, no more outflow occurs, and the entire hernia comes up to arterial pressure. When the hernia is at arterial pressure, no more arterial blood can enter, and there is no more blood flow to the contents of the hernia! As you can imagine, if a vital organ, such as a loop of bowel, is in the hernia, this is an emergency.

This same process of venous occlusion, followed by rise in pressure and cessation of arterial flow, can occur when a finger with a ring is injured. The ring must be removed of course! We have special ring cutters in the ER for that very purpose.

Sometimes I am able to gently but firmly, after giving some pain medication, reduce (return the contents to their proper place) a stubborn hernia. If I cannot reduce the hernia, I promptly call the surgeon. In my experience, general surgeons are especially good at reducing hernias, and this is likely due to their greater understanding of their anatomy. If the surgeon cannot reduce the hernia, and some will not elect to try if I have failed, the patient is taken to the operating room for emergent surgical reduction and repair.

If you suddenly have a bulging hernia that will not reduce, there is no time to waste. Go straight to the ER.

If a loop of bowel is caught in an incarcerated hernia, signs of bowel obstruction often occur (see the "Abdominal Pain" chapter) and these include vomiting, abdominal distension, and severe intermittent pain. Pain and tenderness of the hernia itself are typical with an incarcerated hernia, though the degree of pain is variable.

Other types of hernia are not visible externally, and a hiatal (a.k.a. hiatus) hernia is one of them. A hiatal hernia is when a part of the stomach protrudes through the diaphragm (the thin muscular layer that separates the abdomen from the chest) at the place where the esophagus passes through into the chest. A hiatal hernia can go unnoticed, or it can cause gastroesophageal reflux or pain.

Rarely, a hiatal hernia can become incarcerated, which can cause severe pain, vomiting, and serious problems. Before CT was commonly used in the diagnosis of abdominal pain, I admitted one of these to the surgeon. The best I could do was say, "I can't give you an exact diagnosis, but something is very wrong in her abdomen, and it seems surgical." The surgeon stopped by the ER two days later to tell me the story of how he diagnosed the incarcerated hiatal hernia and let me know that the patient was recovering well after her surgery.

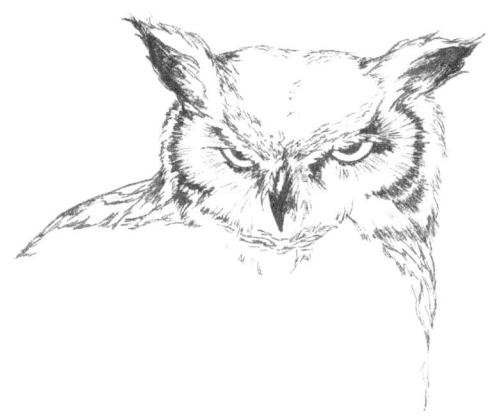

Chapter 26
Hypertension (High Blood Pressure)

It's the terror of knowing, What this world is about…
Watching some good friends Screaming, "let me out!"

—from the song "Under Pressure," by David Bowie

As an emergency physician, I see many patients who are worried about their blood pressure. The commonest situation I see is when a person comes to the ER after seeing some high numbers on their home blood-pressure cuff. Most of these patients are having no symptoms and are, of course, already on medications for their blood pressure. One of my colleagues once said, "The best way to treat this problem is to ask to see their blood-pressure cuff—and then gift it to a medical student!"

Yesterday I cared for a seventy-seven-year-old lady named Alice who called the ambulance when she took her blood pressure for the third time during an hour and found that it had continued to rise. He first reading was 142/92. She became a bit worried, and a few minutes later checked it again. It had risen to 147/94. This made her worry quite a bit more, and she "walked around the house a few times" to see if that would help. She noticed that the neighbor's cat was stalking birds at her feeder on the deck, and she shooed it away. As she turned to go back in the house, she saw that a cedar shingle had blown off her roof, which upset her because it made her remember that her husband had been putting off cleaning the gutters. (As she told the story, I noted her husband wince and look down.) She brought the shingle in to him (he was watching football) and had it join him on the couch! She then went into the kitchen, and her blood pressure was up to 158/105. She became even more worried and called 911.

The paramedics put her on the monitor, gave her an aspirin, spoke calming words, and brought her to the ER. By the time she arrived, her blood pressure was 138/82, which is within normal range. I reassured her that her pressure was now fine and promised to watch her for a bit on the monitor. Alice had recently had a thorough heart workup and was given a clean bill of health by the cardiologist. She was on two different blood-pressure medications, and her blood pressure had actually been a bit low at times recently. After half an hour of uneventful monitoring—and lunch—she went home. Worrying about blood pressure can definitely increase blood pressure!

A blood pressure is considered elevated if it is higher than 140/90. The commonest cause of high blood pressure by far is "idiopathic," which means "nobody knows why." Another name for hypertension without an identifiable cause is essential hypertension. Hypertension is genetic (inherited) and is commoner in some races than others.

What is Blood Pressure?

There is no big secret to how blood pressure works. The numbers represent actual pressures in centimeters of water. The same number equals millimeters of mercury (since mercury is about ten times denser than water). A blood pressure of 120 is pressure enough to push water up a tube against gravity to a height of 120 centimeters.

Understanding the two numbers is worthwhile. The first number is the "systolic" blood pressure, and the second is the "diastolic" blood pressure. Systole is the contraction/pumping part of the heart cycle, and diastole is the relaxation phase. The maximum (contraction) amount of pressure is the systolic pressure, and the relaxation pressure during the cycle is the diastolic pressure. The pressure in the arterial system obviously does not drop to zero in normal circumstances, but averages between the two pressures. Even while the heart relaxes, the elasticity of the arteries maintains pressure and forward flow. "Mean arterial pressure" is a function of averaging the two pressures, with a preference of two-thirds given to the relaxation phase pressure, since more time is spent in relaxation than in contraction.

Some causes of high blood pressure are treatable, and these should be excluded by your primary doctor before medical treatment is started. One cause we are taught to look for in medical school is "renal artery stenosis." When the renal arteries are narrowed, the kidneys sense less blood pressure and release a chemical that raises the body's overall blood pressure. If the narrowing is repaired, the pressure returns to normal. Lifestyle can affect blood pressure. Smoking and obesity will raise blood pressure. Some people, especially the elderly and those of African American ancestry, tend to be "salt sensitive," and increasing salt intake will increase blood pressure.

There are usually no noticeable symptoms to alert a person that their blood pressure is high. Blood pressure is not like tire pressure. If tire pressure is too high, there will definitely be uneven wear and at worst a "blowout" coming in the future. A person can live a long and perfectly normal life with elevated blood pressure, and a mildly elevated blood pressure will not only be unnoticed, but will cause no harm on a short-term, and possibly long-term, basis. A healthy person's systolic blood pressure tends to increase with age as the arteries stiffen. Since the arteries are less "stretchable," the force of the heart is pushing against a harder system when it contracts, and the result is a higher (systolic/top) number.

If you have high blood pressure—and it should be confirmed on several office visits at least—treatment can reduce lifetime risks of some common problems, including heart attack and stroke.

Hypertension Treatment

How effective is treating hypertension? This is an interesting question. In medical practice, we often use the phrase "number needed to treat." The number needed to treat answers the question: "How many people will I need to treat for a certain number of years to prevent a particular problem?" The number needed to treat with lice (pesticide shampoo) medicine to cure lice is one. If you apply the pesticide properly, the lice are killed. The number of people older than sixty who need to be treated for mild hypertension daily for five years to prevent one stroke is harder to calculate, but it is about 170. In other words, since 170 people times 5 years equals 835 person-years, a single person would need to be treated for about 835 years to prevent a stroke. Clearly, if you have mild hypertension, missing a day of your medicine is not worth losing sleep over!

When I was explaining this principle to Alice, in an effort to tell her she would not "have a blow out," I used an example. I asked her the question, "If two people had a mildly elevated blood pressure like yours, and one received treatment and the other did not, what would happen?" Alice answered in a typical manner. She said, "The one who wasn't treated wouldn't live as long." Every patient I ask seems to have the same impression. The more accurate answer would be, "In most cases there would be no difference."

Controlling high blood pressure is a big business for doctors and drug companies. Managing blood pressure is straightforward—and rewarding—because the right medications definitely lower the number. It feels good, as a physician, to "get the job done." Ah, if only it were that simple!

Is there a downside to taking blood-pressure medication? Absolutely! Every year I see people who fall and have other accidents because their blood pressure gets too low, causing lightheadedness. Every emergency physician has sutured scalp and facial lacerations and treated fractures that occurred as a direct result of falls caused by a treated blood pressure that went too low.

I have also seen strokes that occurred when blood pressure was lowered. Sometimes more pressure is needed to force blood through narrowed arteries, and if the carotid arteries (main neck arteries) are narrowed, dropping the pressure to them…well, you can see. Twenty years ago we treated high blood pressure more aggressively in stroke and head injury than we do today. The trend today is toward preserving blood flow and decreasing brain oxygen demand, rather than decreasing pressure.

Choosing a Blood Pressure Medicine

When choosing an initial blood-pressure medication, there are a number of options, and one is often likely to fit a particular person better than others. If you must take a medicine, why not choose one that will make you feel better? For a patient who is salt sensitive and tends toward holding water and leg swelling, for example, a diuretic might be ideal. A diuretic will decrease the leg swelling as a comfortable side benefit. For the person who feels tense or who experiences frequent palpitations, a "beta blocker" might be a good choice. Beta blockers are sometimes used by people who give presentations in front of groups. A beta blocker, by stopping some of the "adrenaline effect," makes a person's body feel calm. On the down side, a beta blocker can affect the heart in the same way a "governor" acts on an engine. The beta blocker will decrease the ability of the heart to speed up and thus may decrease a person's "horsepower" and physical performance. On the good side, a beta blocker might prevent a heart attack by decreasing the heart's oxygen demand.

There are a number of other medications as well, and you should, if your blood pressure is proven to be higher than ideal, discuss all the options with your doctor.

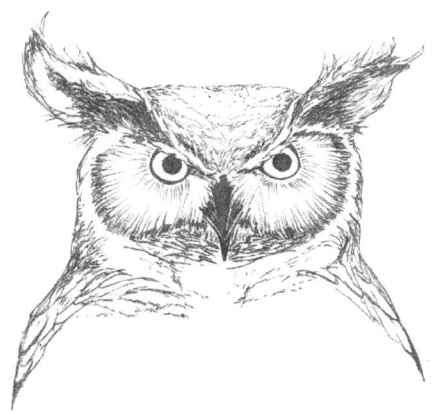

Chapter 27
Infection

A child who is protected from all controversial ideas is as vulnerable as a child who is protected from every germ. The infection, when it comes—and it will come—may overwhelm the system, be it the immune system, or the belief system.

—Jane Smiley

Throughout this book we discuss infection repeatedly. Some specific infections need to be covered in their respective chapters. In this chapter, we will cover some general concepts. Infections are one of the most treatable problems we have and the most likely problem—

other than injury—that you will encounter in your first fifty years of life.

My medical boxes are certainly much more than first-aid kits. They contain oral, topical, and injectable (parenteral) antibiotics. I have used the antibiotics over the years to successfully treat many friends, my family, our dogs, horses, birds, fish, and, just last month, our milk goat, Jean.

Signs of Infection

The classic signs of infection were first described about 2000 years ago. They were (and remain today); dolor (pain), calor (heat), rubor (redness), and tumor (swelling).

Sometimes infection is obvious, and sometimes subtle. While an infected, oozing wound may be hard to miss, a bladder infection in an elderly patient has led many a physician on a "merry chase."

When a previously healthy creature (adult, child, or animal) suddenly begins to be less active, to lose weight, or to otherwise decline, infection should be considered. If a reason for decline is not discovered on investigation, treating for bacterial infection while giving general support will often lead to recovery. Some of my fellow physicians will accuse me of heresy for that last statement, since it is best to know what infection is being treated, but I will persist and argue that what I want to see is survival.

Fishing Break!

I love fly fishing, but if the fish aren't biting on flies, I'll switch to spoons, spinners, or (heresy!) even bait. During college at Washington State University, I was invited to fish the Grande Rhonde River for steelhead. Some excellent fly fishermen invited me when they learned I owned a bunch of fly rods and tied my own trout flies. We all started fishing, and after four hours of flogging the water with every fly in our boxes, we still hadn't had a bite. I had my ultralight spinning rod in the trunk and, with a small black "Roostertail" spinner, made a cast into the deep pool I thought was the best looking water I had fished all morning. "Bang!" A smashing strike, and an eight-pound steelhead leapt clear of the water. After a long battle, one of my (now ex) fishing buddies helped net the fish. I put the spinning rod back in the trunk, but after another hour of fly casting, couldn't resist pulling it out again. On the second cast, I hooked an eleven-pounder, which I followed downstream almost to the Snake River before gently removing the barbless hook from her mouth and releasing her. I admire fly-fishing purists, but I also love catching fish.

In the same spirit, if I am treating a seriously ill patient, and I can't find a source of infection, but suspect one, that person won't leave my ER without a bunch of strong antibiotics in their blood.

Causes of infection include bacteria, viruses, fungus, and parasites. Of these, our current medications are least effective against viruses.

Infections can be obvious in location, or they can be systemic (found throughout the body). Some of the worst infections start out in a particular spot and then spread either to adjacent areas or to the blood. Overwhelming blood-borne infection is known as "sepsis."

In the "Ear Pain" chapter, I stated that an otitis media (middle-ear infection) is "not considered an acceptable (source) cause of fever." A very rare ear infection can spread to the mastoid bone (the hard, thick bone behind the ear) and surrounding soft tissues, or can move into the fluid that surrounds the brain, and then a fever is almost certain to occur. Bacterial infections that become systemic (moving throughout the body) are very bad indeed.

How Colds Cause Discomfort

Some infections are always systemic. The common cold and influenza are examples. These viral infections often cause fever. You will notice/recall that with these infections there are multiple symptoms, in many parts of the body. The flu or a cold (there are a virtually limitless number of viruses and variations of viruses that cause cold symptoms, and influenza is one of them) often causes a sore throat, body aches, cough, runny nose/congestion, and headache. These symptoms are caused not so much by the virus as by the body's attempts at killing the virus. In effect, the body is the battlefield.

Drugs that stop the body's inflammatory response to a cold reduce the symptoms of the cold. Removing some inflammatory tissue, such as the tonsils, will reduce the severity of future sore throats by removing "the field of battle."

Picture this. Look at the door of the room in which you are currently reading. What if suddenly a hundred soldiers with guns and grenades came to the door and started entering the room? Pretty scary, eh? Now, say they are only one-inch tall. One approaches your ankle and fires his rifle at it. You feel a slight tickle as the bullet bounces off, and you go back to reading. Eventually they give up and go away, leaving very little mud on the floor, since their feet are only a few millimeters long. Now, what if instead you yelled, "Soldiers! We're under attack!" and grabbed your shotgun and started shooting. You would blow holes in the floor, bust a few pipes, possibly even damage several other rooms in the house. After you depleted your fifty rounds of bird shot, there would still be a bunch of the little fellows left to call in more forces.

In the case of a cold, the house is your body, and the shotgun is your body's immune system. That is how a cold causes discomfort!

Whether or not a person with an intact immune system catches a cold depends on a combination of how much experience their body has with the particular virus, how heavily they are exposed, and the virulence (aggression, rate of growth, ability to spread and cause infection) of the particular virus.

The main reason colds are more common in the winter is not that the cold weather causes people to get sick, but that the cold weather causes people to congregate indoors, where they are more likely to spread a virus from person to person.

Virus on a Plane! How the Flu Spreads and How to Avoid it

Flying on an airplane is a great way to catch a cold or the flu. Recently my family and I flew to Hawaii, a six-hour flight from Seattle. There were enough seats across the middle section of row number 19 to allow my whole family and one additional business traveler to sit there. The businessman was in his mid-thirties and obviously had a bad cold or the flu. He was coughing a lot, sneezing regularly, and blowing his nose loud and hard into tissue several times each hour. In short, he was spreading viral particles like crazy. I sat closest to him, and he was rubbing my left elbow as we "wrestled" for the armrest in the narrow seats. My wife, Erin, was on my right, with my daughter and two sons to her right. Riley, my nine-year old daughter, was on her immediate right, followed by six-year-old Drake and thirteen-year-old Konrad. The incubation period for colds and the flu varies from three to eleven days, so I could look forward to a miserable vacation if I or any of my family members were to contract the virus.

In this situation, I was the closest to the source of the potential infection. Six hours is a long flight, and it was hard to resist the urge to meet the fellow. I fought the urge, leaning toward my wife, for quite a while. Should I meet him and shake his hand? His hands were obviously covered with the virus, so probably not a good idea. I said "bless you" when he sneezed, and he nodded. We shared a few words to alleviate the awkwardness of sitting next to a complete stranger for six hours. I turned up several of the air vents overhead to create a "positive pressure" situation, hopefully causing a flow of air toward him from our direction.

In this case, because I was closest to the source, I was likely to have the greatest exposure. I am also, however, very resistant to most viral infections, having contracted dozens during med school. I also had diagnosed dozens of cases of the much-publicized swine flu in my ER during the preceding month. The flu is very virulent, though, and a six-hour exposure is a completely different level of exposure than seeing a patient for ten minutes. I consciously resisted the urge to rub my eyes.

My wife, being second closest, would have the next highest level of exposure. Erin had just recovered from the flu, and at this time H1N1 (swine flu) was the primary virus in the Seattle area. It was likely the man was suffering from that same virus, and thus Erin was probably immune. The kids were farther from the source and had been heavily exposed to mom, thus either gaining immunity or proving they already had it. That is a lot of variables to consider, isn't it? The bottom line: none of us caught the virus, and we had a great vacation.

When the person next to you on an airplane sneezes, it is almost impossible to avoid breathing some of the viral particles. Luckily the body has a series of mechanical (physical) defenses that reduces exposure before the cellular immune system (white blood cells and antibody, which we have discussed and which are important enough to go over again) comes into play. Some of the viral particles you breathe don't make it past the nose. Most of them are trapped in the mucous layers and subsequently swallowed with the saliva into the stomach, where they are mostly destroyed by stomach acid. Of those that make it past the stomach acid, most are destroyed by the immunity within the intestines, which, as a potential "portal of entry" are heavily patrolled by the body's defenses.

Whether to blow one's nose or to sniffle and swallow in this situation is a question worth pondering. If viral particles from your neighbor are trapped in the nose, blowing the nose will externalize some of them, but will also force some of them into the sinuses and passages to the eyes and ears (nasolacrimal duct and Eustachian tubes), where they can enter sensitive, permeable tissue. Sniffling may allow exposure of other sensitive tissues of the throat and posterior pharynx before the mucous reaches the acid of the stomach, where most of the viral or bacterial particles will be destroyed.

Rubbing the eyes should definitely be avoided, as infection can easily enter from hand-to-eye contact. Forming the habit of not touching one's face after shaking lots of hands at a meeting is a good idea. Wash your hands after such contact.

A viral particle does not live forever outside of its host, and some die on the skin before they can enter the body. The skin itself is a formidable barrier, chemically and physically designed to be hostile to invaders in most circumstances.

Bacterial Infection

Bacterial infections are different from viral infections. A strep throat, for example, is an infection of the throat only. The fever the infection causes will create overall discomfort, but a runny nose and cough do not generally occur, as they usually do with a viral infection. The lymph nodes of the neck will swell as the body fights to prevent the spread of the bacterial infection, and the tonsils swell as they are affected.

Knowing the difference between a cold and a bacterial infection will save you many office and ER visits. Antibiotics work well on bacterial infections, but do not cure viral infections. Furthermore, antibiotics can cause diarrhea, allergic reactions, and other problems.

Antibiotic overuse encourages increasing numbers of antibiotic-resistant bacteria. Everyone is exposed to antibiotic-resistant bacteria these days, but in the absence of antibiotics, these bacteria are at a disadvantage. For a bacterium to be antibiotic resistant, it must carry additional genetic material. If there are no antibiotics around, this additional material is just "excess baggage," and the normal bacteria will have the reproductive advantage. If there are antibiotics present, however, the antibiotic-resistant bacteria have the advantage. In the continued presence of antibiotics, they will eventually predominate.

If they then cause an infection, the resistant infection will be harder to cure.

Most colds cause a cough, but a bacterial infection of the lungs (pneumonia/bronchitis) is limited to the lungs in the same way that strep throat is limited to the throat. Once again, the fever and bodily stress can make one feel generally poor, but the pain is in the chest, coughing and sputum production (depending on the type of infection) are prominent, and there is no accompanying sore throat, congestion of the nose, and so on.

Sinusitis Can Have Many Causes

Sinusitis is common, if we take "sinusitis" to mean inflammation of the sinuses; however, bacterial (treatable with antibiotics) sinusitis is much rarer. In this area, the commonest story I hear is from a patient who has been suffering from "sinusitis" for months. Jamie, a twenty-nine-year-old legal assistant I treated last month, was typical. She had been suffering from sinus congestion and headaches that were worse when she bent over to file documents (something legal assistants do a lot of, I inferred!). She also had nasal drainage, and it was sometimes green or brown in color.

Jamie initially asked me for a "stronger" antibiotic. She explained that she had first been given amoxicillin. Amoxicillin is currently the first antibiotic recommended for sinusitis and is usually prescribed for ten days. After ten days she was no better. She was next prescribed Augmentin, which is amoxicillin mixed with another antibiotic called clavulinic acid. That combination will defeat many antibiotic-resistant bacteria. After ten days of Augmentin, during which time she had experienced stomach upset and diarrhea (not uncommon with Augmentin), she was still no better. Returning to her doctor, she was placed on a very different antibiotic, known as azithromycin, in the form of a "Z-pack." Taken for five days, but remaining in the body for at least twice that long, azithromycin is relatively new and quite effective against a broad range of bacteria. After five days she was no better. When she called her doctor, he advised her that the azithromycin would be active in her body for at least another week and that she should be patient.

She came to my ER at the end of that next week. Her sinusitis involved the sinus cavities of her lower forehead (frontal sinuses) on both sides, as well as those under her eyes (maxillary sinuses) on both sides of her face. She had not had a fever, and she explained that the problem began when she took her new job. I asked her about her new place of work. It was a private legal office in a remodeled Victorian house in the old downtown district. During the first days of her new job, she smelled a lot of "musty odors," but had not noticed it since. Probably her nasal congestion had decreased her sense of smell.

I explained to Jamie that she was not suffering from bacterial sinusitis, but rather from allergic sinusitis. All the antibiotics in the world will not cure allergic sinusitis. We discussed the possibility of cleaning up the old building and of finding a new job. Jamie liked her job, and since it was a new legal practice and not yet busy, she had a lot of time to clean up the place. I started her on a combination of pseudoephedrine to decongest her nasal passages and sinuses and a short course of oral prednisone to knock down the inflammation, followed by a twice-daily nasal anti-inflammatory spray to maintain the anti-inflammatory effect without the systemic (whole body) effect of the oral steroid. Five days later one of my colleagues in the ER took a call from Jamie. She was "one hundred percent better, and very thankful."

Often we see a big increase in allergic sinusitis in the spring, when flowers are blooming and airborne pollen counts are up. I probably see about one hundred cases of allergic sinusitis each year and maybe one case of bacterial sinusitis per year. I refer the bacterial cases to the ENT (otolaryngologist) after initiating treatment. A bacterial sinusitis is most often localized to a single sinus—"Right here under my right cheek, Doc"—is often accompanied by fever, and can be a very serious problem indeed. Bacterial sinusitis in diabetic and other immune-compromised patients is a special cause for concern.

Vaccination and Resistance

Earlier we discussed the resistance to infection and how that resistance varies from person to person. Once a person has been infected by a particular pathogen, and his or her body has created specific antibodies, the person's body is ready to recognize and neutralize that particular infection. If a long time passes without exposure to the infection, the acquired immunity will slowly decrease. If enough time passes without another exposure (reason to maintain those specific antibodies), immunity may decrease to the point where infection is once again possible.

Vaccination is a way of educating the body to recognize and neutralize a particular bacteria or virus without actually being exposed to the full strength (and dangers) of an infection. The pathogen (bacteria or virus) is characterized by a particular surface texture (particular antigen), which must be recognized to be effectively attacked. White cells called lymphocytes make antibodies to fit a given texture. When an antibody that fits that texture finds it, it sticks to the pathogen, allowing the body's warrior white cells, known as phagocytes, to recognize and envelop it. Once inside the phagocyte, the enemy is destroyed.

Everyone has a bunch of different "clones" of lymphocytes waiting around, ready to create an antibody to a particular infection if needed. If you have already had chicken pox, for example, you have a clone of lymphocytes that make an antibody to chicken pox floating around in your blood all the time. If you are exposed again to a small amount of chicken-pox virus, the antibody you already have will stick to the virus, neutralizing it and allowing the phagocytes to eat it up. Being exposed will trigger more of the chicken-pox clone lymphocytes to be created, and a greater amount of chicken-pox antibody to be made. If you are not exposed to any chicken pox for many years, your number of chicken-pox lymphocytes will decrease, as will the amount of chicken-pox antibody in your blood. Immunity can thus decrease, and if it decreases enough and if the exposure to chicken pox is large enough to overwhelm the amount of immunity present before the system can get revved up, infection can occur.

An antibody titer can be measured to test the strength of a person's immunity to a particular infection. This is a blood test, and a result is usually not available for at least several days. My level of chicken pox antibody was tested at the start of my residency training to ensure that I retained enough resistance to avoid active infection. This testing was required because chicken pox can cause birth defects if contracted by a pregnant woman, and I could expect to care for many pregnant women during my residency. Even though I'd had chicken pox when I was four years old, I still had a high titer of antibodies when I was tested at thirty years old. If my resistance had fallen to a level where I might catch chicken pox, a vaccine would have been given to "boost my immunity," thus protecting my patients.

Vaccines are made up of either a live, weakened (attenuated) infectious agent or material (antigen) from a killed infectious agent. The hepatitis B vaccine is made up of the outer layer (surface antigen) of hepatitis virus, but no material from inside the virus (core). If a person is actually infected by hepatitis B, they develop antibodies to both the outside and inside of the virus. Picture a battle between a bunch of viruses and a bunch of white blood cells, with pieces of mutilated virus flying in all directions! A person can be tested to see if they have resistance to hepatitis B. If they are found to have antibodies to the surface, but not the core, they got their resistance from the vaccine. If they have antibodies to both the surface and core (viral "guts" strewn about the battlefield), they developed their resistance by being infected.

Medical Wisdom

Chicken pox (varicella) is an interesting infection and illustrates some important points. When I was a boy, there was no active vaccination program targeting chicken pox, but now there is. How good is the immunity conferred by the vaccine? Is it as good as the immunity a person gets by actually fighting the infection? A titer can be drawn to test the level of antibody, but we do not yet know the long-term efficacy of the vaccine.

Vaccines are a hot topic among the lay public and self-educated/pseudomedical people, but there is very little controversy among physicians and scientists. There is no scientific evidence that vaccines cause autism, birth defects, cerebral palsy, hyperactivity, or any of the other rumored effects that people are worried about. It is clear that vaccines have eradicated many serious diseases and that their benefit to society massively outweighs their downside. I have never met a practicing physician who did not advocate routine vaccination.

Some reaction to a vaccine is expected. It is the reaction that creates the immune response. Localized pain and swelling are common. Vaccines should always be given under medical supervision, in case an allergic reaction occurs.

"Herd immunity" is achieved when the majority of people/animals in a group are immune. People in our society who refuse to have vaccinations and/or refuse to have their children vaccinated are relying on the fact that the rest of the "herd" of humans is immune and that they will therefore not be exposed. This becomes a problem, however, when people agree among themselves not to be vaccinated. We had an outbreak of pertussis (whooping cough) on the south end of our island last year. The south end of the island is known to harbor a large number of free thinkers, whereas the north end is known to be more conventional. Vaccination is conventional, since all the doctors on the island recommend it. Many of the free thinkers send their children to the same schools, and the outbreak occurred at those schools on the south end of the island.

Chapter 27 Infection

Going to the ER with a cold is not required in most cases, but there are times when you should definitely go, or bring your child. The commonest reasons to need emergency care for a viral infection are dehydration and shortness of breath. Dehydration can occur faster with a fever, and vomiting and diarrhea contribute. Signs of dehydration include dry mouth and thirstiness, increased heart rate at rest, cooler hands and feet, and slowed capillary refill of the skin. The heart rate increases as the volume of blood is decreased during dehydration. Less blood is pumped with each heartbeat, so more beats are needed per minute to get enough blood moving. Cooler hands and feet result from the body's ability to use the decreased blood volume most effectively: by decreasing the flow to the arms and legs, more blood is available for vital organ systems.

Judging Hydration

Capillary refill is what occurs when you push on your skin and watch it become pale and then pink up again. Pushing on the skin or nail bed forces blood out of the small blood vessels known as capillaries, which then returns to them at a varying rate. Capillary refill is easier to see in some places than others. I usually look at a child's fingers and toes, and then compare the speed of pinking up with the face and ear (which I tug on gently while checking for ear infection). The one time when capillary refill can be misleading is with very serious life-threatening infection (sepsis), which causes failure of the body's normal control of blood-vessel tone and thus blood pressure.

Test your capillary refill by pressing hard on the skin of your hand with the opposite index finger. Either the back of your hand or the palm will work. If you do not wear colored nail polish, the pink nail bed works well. As I stand here typing, in the warm house, my capillary refill is less than one second. Two seconds and under is normal. Above two seconds means the body is decreasing the blood flow to the extremities.

Medical Wisdom

In a child with a cold, a few episodes of vomiting and a few episodes of diarrhea can be tolerated without dehydration. If vomiting and diarrhea continue for more than a day or so, though, signs of dehydration can be expected. Once the vomiting is controlled, it is usually possible to maintain hydration, despite diarrheal losses. A single dose of an antiemetic such as Zofran in the emergency department can break the vomiting cycle and allow a child to rehydrate by drinking.

Viral infections of the gastrointestinal tract are the commonest cause of diarrhea worldwide. In the United States, rotavirus is the commonest cause of severe diarrhea and vomiting in infants and children. As of 2006 an effective vaccine for rotavirus has been available. This vaccine is probably worthwhile because the vomiting and especially the diarrhea can be severe and usually lasts for three to eight days. We will talk about rotavirus more in the "Pediatric Problems" chapter.

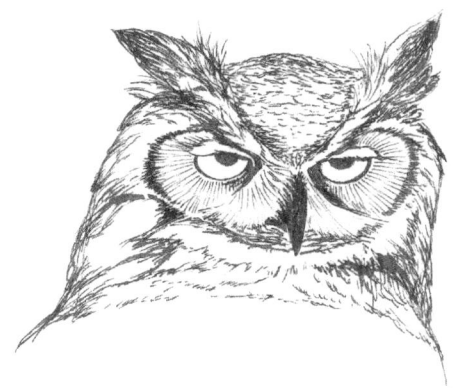

Chapter 28
Jaundice

All looks yellow to a jaundiced eye.

—Alexander Pope, English poet, circa 1720

The development of a yellow skin color is known as jaundice. Jaundice can be most noticeable when it affects the whites (conjunctiva) of the eyes. When jaundice comes on gradually, a spouse may not notice until it is pronounced. Jaundice is caused either by an obstruction of the outflow from the liver or by failure of the liver to eliminate bilirubin fast enough.

Jaundice is a serious symptom and should prompt an immediate visit to a doctor if it occurs in a person who has not had it regularly.

Jaundice with an illness and pain in the liver (right upper abdomen—the location of gallstone-caused pain, as we discussed in the "Abdominal Pain" chapter) can be caused by infectious hepatitis. The word hepatitis simply means inflammation of the liver and can be caused by many things besides infection.

Well-known infectious causes of hepatitis include hepatitis A, which is contracted by the "oral fecal" route, often by consuming shellfish or seafood from contaminated water. Hepatitis A causes a serious illness and jaundice if contracted as an adult. In third-world countries with poorer sanitation, it is very prevalent; the majority of children contract it with minimal resultant symptoms and then are immune to further infection. Hepatitis A, unlike other forms of hepatitis, does not become chronic and does not cause postinfection mortality.

When I was in my early twenties, my father encouraged me to get the hepatitis B vaccine, which I then received. He was concerned that since I was a commercial diver, working around boats in marinas, I would be exposed to pollution and infected with hepatitis. You now know that the vaccine for hepatitis B would not protect against the form of hepatitis to which a diver would be exposed, which is hepatitis A. My father was an orthopedist, but meant well.

Your doctor will run a test on the bilirubin to determine if the jaundice is caused by bilirubin that has been through the liver and then forced back into the blood, or if it has not been through the liver. This will help determine if the problem is one of obstruction of bilirubin elimination or of increased production.

Jaundice should not be ignored, as it is often a sign of a serious problem that can be treated, if caught in time. "Do not let a loved one sleep on yellowed sheets."

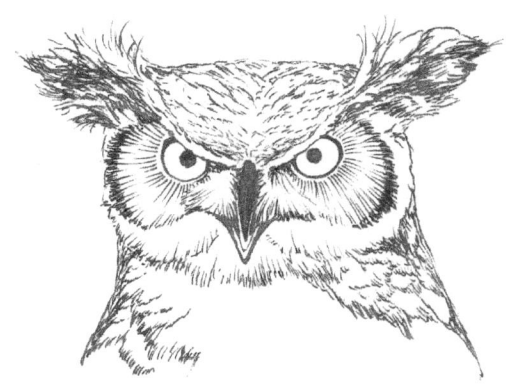

Chapter 29
Joint Pain

I don't deserve this award, but I have arthritis and I don't deserve that either.

—*Jack Benny*

This chapter overlaps somewhat with the "Extremity Pain without Trauma" chapter, but some of these problems are very common and deserve thorough coverage.

Joints—the places where different bones come together—are coated with smoother, softer material known as cartilage. Cartilage is rubbery and tough. You have certainly encountered some when eating chicken. Some joints have no additional padding, and others give the smooth, firm cartilage attached to the end of the bone some assistance. The knee, for example, has additional padding called the meniscus. A meniscal tear is a common knee injury that results in blood within the knee joint, pain, and sometimes a popping or locking of the joint as this additional pad moves out of place and blocks the joint's movement.

I don't remember having joint pain for no apparent reason until my forties. Now I wake up with it every day. My wife does, too, and so does everyone I talk to. From this, and from what my patients tell me, I gather that a certain amount of joint pain is expected as we age.

The type of aching joint pain and stiffness that everyone experiences past the age of thirty or so is known as osteoarthritis, which is the inflammation and pain that results from wear and tear. Injuries can speed normal arthritis by causing misalignment and abnormal stresses on the joints. When a joint is damaged, the body tries to repair the damage and "clean up the rough edges." Joints are further damaged by the inflammation during that repair, in the same way that the inflammation in a smoker's lung destroys the lung tissue.

Does hard use speed arthritis? Will a marathon runner's knees need replacement sooner than the average "desk jockey"? That question is not simple to answer. One of the recurrent themes as you read this text is "the body will adapt." The marathon runner has nicely toned muscles holding those hard-worked joints in nice alignment, whereas the desk jockey's soft muscles allow the joints to be sloppy, misaligned, and prone to injury. The runner has improved balance and lighter weight, factors that decrease joint wear and prevent injury. The runner's increased bone density can prevent a fracture or other injury and therefore prevent the joint problems associated with that injury.

Everyone is called upon to perform physically on occasion, and when the athlete gets the phone call, "I need your help to move," he or she is better able to handle a hard day of carrying stuff up and down the stairs. "Weekend warriors" are prone to injury.

Chapter 29 Joint Pain

Studies have been done to determine if lots of running is damaging to the joints. I have reviewed many of these in the quest for the answer. I can find no evidence that running, unless acute injury occurs, causes either premature wearing out of the joints or joint damage.

Since arthritis is caused by inflammation, can anti-inflammatory pain medications actually help as not just a pain reducer, but as a cure for the inflammation? That is also a great question. Ibuprofen is a commonly used nonsteroidal anti-inflammatory, as is aspirin. Aspirin and ibuprofen certainly reduce joint pain, but how do they do it? If they do it by actually stopping the inflammation, then they should, in theory, reduce joint damage and make the joints last longer. This is not as clear cut as it might seem at first inspection, however. The inflammatory process is needed to rebuild, as well as to tear down. Good studies show that broken bones heal slower when ibuprofen is given during the healing period. I spent quite a bit of time trying to come up with a clear consensus on this question, and "the jury is still out." Right now using anti-inflammatory pain medications as a prophylactic against the aging process is not recommended.

In recent years there has been a movement toward the use of oral supplements to help joint pain. Glucosamine and chondroitin are effective when used for joint pain, for some people, and do little, if any, good for others. Initially when I heard of the oral supplements, I didn't see how they could work (beyond the placebo effect). Dr. Robert Tait of Davis, California, explained a more plausible mechanism of action to me. Bob is a superb scientist, with substantial discoveries and insight to his credit. As he explained, if the inflammation of the joints is caused by the body's attack on its own cartilage, the intake of cartilage (chondroitin is cartilage) and the constant exposure to this cartilage and its components could desensitize the body's immune system to cartilage. If the body is less sensitive to joint tissue, it may be able to "ignore" the joints and thus cause less joint inflammation and damage. I thanked Bob, who is also one of the fittest and most active people I know, for this insight.

When a joint is just plain worn out, replacement is sometimes an option. Knee and hip replacements are the commonest and can sometimes work miracles. If you are heading toward a knee or hip replacement, or know someone who is, the best advice is, "Those who walk in for the replacement walk out." What I mean by that is if a person develops severe knee pain and spends weeks or months in a wheelchair/not walking before the replacement, recovery will be difficult. Replacing the joint is great, but all the muscles are still original issue! Some patients expect that the replacement will eliminate their pain, and they are often surprised at first. The pain you have after surgery will be different, but very real. Be sure you have adequate pain medicine to help you overcome the postsurgical pain and to help you get back on your feet as soon as possible.

If you have been fighting the battle against osteoarthritis and have increased the aspirin/ibuprofen/other pain medications to their highest doses and still have a lot of pain, seeing the orthopedic surgeon may be a good idea. It is better to walk (or at least limp!) in for that appointment, too. Increase your activity during the weeks before the replacement, so your muscles will be toned and strong, and continue on the strength training as well. Joint replacement can be easily done under regional or spinal anesthesia, and you should be given that option.

We discussed some of the autoimmune joint problems in the earlier chapter. Osteoarthritis is different from rheumatoid arthritis, which is more debilitating and can strike in youth. Rheumatoid arthritis (RA) generally causes marked swelling of the affected joint, and the symptoms can be migratory.

The first example of rheumatoid arthritis I was unfortunate enough to witness struck my childhood friend Pete. We were on a camping/falconry trip to Montana, and we camped alongside the Missouri

Chapter 29 Joint Pain

River. Pete was a very active person and a natural athlete. He could sit on the ground with his legs out in front of him, put his fingertips on the ground by his hips, and go straight into a handstand without apparent effort. Pete could also climb trees much better than I and was physically tireless. I had just turned eighteen years old at the time, and Pete seemed much older to me, and much wiser, since he was about twenty. We were camping on a small meadow beside the Missouri River in Montana. When we awoke in the morning, Pete showed me his right elbow and said it "really hurt." I could see that the elbow was swollen and red. Pete said that if he hooked his thumb in his belt, it felt better. We tried to remember how he might have hurt it, but couldn't come up with an injury. As the day went on it seemed to be about the same. The next day it was much better, and the third day the swelling was gone. Two days later, though, Pete's right knee was swollen and painful. He limped for two days, but then the knee got better, too. After we returned home to California, Pete continued to have joint pain. He was diagnosed with rheumatoid arthritis and has been fighting it ever since. Despite his severe arthritis, Pete makes some of the finest and most intricate leather products for falconry available anywhere.

As a hand surgeon, my father performed some joint replacements for RA patients. He would say when comparing osteoarthritis with rheumatoid, "A person with osteoarthritis wakes up in the morning and says, boy, do my joints ache. Later, on the golf course, he is feeling better. The person with rheumatoid arthritis starts the day feeling better than when he went to sleep, but as the day goes on, the pain gets worse, and soon he is thinking about getting back in bed. The golf course seems too far away to consider."

The Gout

Gouty arthritis is a distinctive problem worth discussing. A high level of uric acid in the blood results in the formation of uric acid crystals in a joint. The classic picture of a patient with gout is a Pickwickian gentleman with his foot on a pillow, the base of the big toe red and throbbing with pain. Even the slightest movement or the weight of the bed sheet on the toe causes severe pain. Motrin or another anti-inflammatory helps the pain during an acute attack, but aspirin should not be used. Weight loss and decreasing meat, seafood, and alcohol in the diet can help to decrease the rate of attacks. There are also medicines to lower the uric acid level.

An infection of a joint is a very serious problem. Sometimes the infection comes from an injury that punctures the joint, and sometimes the infection comes from another source within the body and finds its way to the joint. The area within a joint contains lubricant known as synovial fluid. There is no direct blood circulation to the joint, and an infection can take over very quickly. An infection in the joint causes massive inflammation and severe pain. A joint infection is a very serious problem, both life threatening and, if not treated quickly by the orthopedic surgeon, very destructive to the joint.

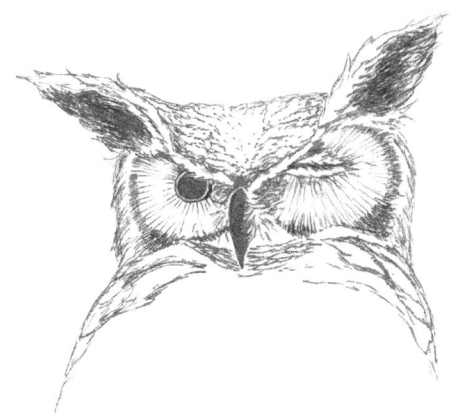

Chapter 30
The Medical Laboratory

The United States is now being dissected in Frankenstein's Laboratory.

—Dr. Laurie Roth, Newswithviews.com, February 20, 2009

If you have ever heard the expressions "Let's send some labs" or "We'll check your urine," then you know what this chapter is about.

During the last twenty years (and more), the medical laboratory has become more and more automated. There are still some manual examinations of specimens, but mostly, blood is squirted into a machine, and the result emerges printed on a slip of paper. Increasingly, the paper is eliminated, and the result is computerized. The machines were once big enough to fill a room, but now are often small enough to be held in a single palm.

One of the potential "problems" with the modern medical lab is that it is very easy to check a lot of things. For every dozen or so things that are checked in a normal person, one (it usually seems like more) thing will come back abnormal. This occurs because all the results are supposed to fall within a "normal range," but like everything else in nature, normal is defined by the observer, and normal encompasses a range of possibilities. "Normal height" for a human, Caucasian male may be between five feet four inches and six feet four inches, but if someone is measured at six feet eight, is that abnormal?

There is also the problem of range of accuracy, which varies and which causes many errors and much variability. If I only check one thing, the chances are good that the measurement will be accurate, but if I check twenty lab values, probably at least one will be affected by an inaccuracy. When blood is drawn in the ER, checking twenty values would be on the low/average side. I make the decision to ignore "abnormal" lab values every time I work.

When I was moonlighting during my emergency medicine residency (lots of doctors do that because residency doesn't pay very well), I worked one or two days a month in a small hospital in the Sierra foothills, where I did twenty-four-hour shifts. When I saw a patient, I would order labs I felt were appropriate, and the results came to me cut out of a larger printout and scotch-taped to a piece of paper. After I had worked there for a while, I got to know the lab personnel. One day the tech suggested I "add a sodium level" to my orders. I asked why and was told that it "might be interesting." I added it, and a minute later received another piece of paper with a scotch-taped cutout that read, "Na – 119." Very interesting indeed! With a sodium of 119, serious changes in brain function are expected, and admission to the hospital is required.

Chapter 30 The Medical Laboratory

After I began treatment and the patient was admitted to the hospital, I visited the "clairvoyant" lab tech. He explained to me that they only had one machine. He showed me how it worked. The machine was about three times as big as a full-sized refrigerator. There was one place up front where the blood was injected into the machine and another where the paper printout emerged. The machine did only one thing: it printed out a comprehensive blood analysis. I would only get the bits of information I asked for, and the patient would only be charged for those tests. All the information was there, though, which explained how I could add a test, after my initial orders, and get the result in a matter of moments!

After that day I would sometimes ask questions like, "Hey, Tim, is there anything else I should know?" or "Give me a little something to go on here, man!" To the average person, a flat fee for labs would seem appropriate in this situation, but billing rules are specific. Sometimes my patients got a very good deal. Other times, a machine error would cause me a lot of extra work and give my patients a chance to read some magazines while waiting.

Other Possible Errors

We go through lots of careful labeling checks to ensure specimens are not mixed up, but a small percentage of errors still occur. If something just doesn't make sense and doesn't correlate with your history or with what you are feeling, rechecking a lab value is a good idea. Things have progressed so far away from the "old days," when the physician himself examined a patient's blood and urine under a microscope, that we often don't even get to look at the blood and urine anymore.

I always try to see the specimen myself. One time I was suspecting a urinary tract infection in a confused, elderly gentleman. He could not make a urine specimen when asked, so I used my ultrasound to look at the bladder. The bladder was quite full, containing what I estimated to be a liter or so of urine. I ordered a Foley catheter (tube in the penis leading to a bag) and watched the urine come out. It was cloudy and foul smelling, obviously infected. The remainder of the liter of urine was drained and a specimen sent to the lab. I started a combination of antibiotics. About twenty minutes later, the urine result returned, and it was as clean as could be! I asked that a repeat be sent. I mentioned the result to the other doctor on duty, and he seemed unimpressed—until a few minutes later when he was surprised by a severely infected urine result in a patient who had no symptoms of infection! We then conferred. He sent a repeat as well, and the new results made more sense. The urines had been accidentally switched!

Patients are often sent to the ER after a phone call from their primary doctor advising them that a lab result came back at a dangerous, abnormal level. If this happens to you, and you are not having symptoms, be sure the test is repeated before any action is taken.

Routine and Screening Tests

Routine laboratory tests do have value, and your primary doctor will discuss which tests should be done and also should explain the potential benefits. Routine testing should be strongly considered if you have a family history of a particular problem. Blood-sugar testing can help detect diabetes. There will likely be no noticeable symptoms of diabetes until the blood sugar is consistently twice the normal level, and by then the body will have suffered some damage. Treatment can be started if diabetes is detected early, and serious complications prevented. High cholesterol can also be detected and treated before problems arise. As cancer markers are isolated and quantified, cancer detection is becoming increasingly effective.

Currently, though, many things are unknown about some of the cancer "markers," so it is important to ask your doctor about the particular marker and what it means. An example of a marker is "prostate-specific antigen," or PSA. Most of you have heard of PSA. Interestingly enough, prostate specific antigen is neither specific to the prostate nor an antigen.

I once had a female patient who asked, "Do I have to worry about prostate cancer—it does run in my family?" I jokingly replied, "No, since only men have prostates!" If she had asked, "Do I have to worry about having an elevated PSA?" my answer would not have been so easy. Even though women do not have a prostate gland, they do have PSA! The best way for her to avoid having an elevated PSA would be to avoid having it tested!

PSA is produced by a number of body tissues, but in men most of it is produced by the prostate. PSA is produced by both normal prostate tissue and by cancerous prostate tissue. Within the prostate, however, there are cells that produce PSA and cells that do not. A cancer of the prostate cells that do not produce PSA will not result in an elevated PSA, and thus some prostate cancers are missed. In the "Urinary Problems" chapter, we will discuss infection of the prostate and benign enlargement of the prostate, which occurs as a man grows older. Both infection and benign (noncancerous) growth raise the PSA. Many prostate biopsies are done each year in response to an elevated PSA, and most do not show cancer. We will, no doubt, have a test that is truly specific for prostate cancer someday.

Next we will discuss some of the commoner laboratory tests, their purposes, and their utility. We will also discuss some problems that are primarily diagnosed by lab result. Some of these problems will have overlapping discussion in other chapters, as well.

When you see a laboratory result sheet, the name of the item tested will be on the left, the value down the center, and the normal range on the right side. Ask your doctor about the importance of the abnormal values. A slightly abnormal value could be either important or of no significance.

The CBC (Complete Blood Count)

The CBC is basically a physical examination and quantification of the blood.

In the chapter on anemia we discussed the hematocrit. The hematocrit is the percent of the blood that is made up of cells (mostly red blood cells) and is a basic piece of data in the CBC. A low hematocrit means you are anemic. We discussed these levels and what they mean to you in the "Anemia" chapter.

The CBC further looks at the cells themselves. The cells are measured and quantified, as well as seen (if the CBC is done or partially done manually). If the red cells are small and low in hemoglobin (iron) as well as low in number, then the patient may have an iron-deficiency anemia. If they are larger than usual, but fewer and make up less of the blood volume, then the anemia may have another cause, such as vitamin deficiency (see the "Anemia" and "Diet and Exercise" chapters). Red blood cells can show signs of injury, which can be caused by a recent transfusion, or of irregularities, such as in sickle-cell disease.

Visual inspection of the red cells may reveal an infection called malaria, transmitted by mosquitoes, which causes an impressive relapsing fever. Visual inspection may also give other clues to diseases such as lead poisoning.

The CBC also evaluates the white blood cell count, breaking it down into the different types of white blood cells. A simple CBC will differentiate between the phagocytes ("engulfing and destroying the enemy" type white cells) and the lymphocytes (antibody makers and immune modulators). In an acute bacterial infection (I am feeling free to speak more like a doctor now since, if you have read this much of the book, you are no longer medically naïve), the phagocytes rise first, and that phenomena is called a "left shift." In an effort to "get the warrior cells out there," even some young cells are sent. These are called "bands." It is sort of like some of America's Revolutionary War: every man was needed, and even some very young men signed on.

Bacteria, being much larger than viruses, are easier for the phagocytes to find and "eat" without help. If the infection is viral, there will be a shift in the other direction as the lymphocytes proliferate so they can produce antibody that can stick to the virus, neutralizing it, and helping it to be detected and engulfed by the warrior cell. If the white blood cell count is elevated and shows a "left shift," a bacterial source of infection should be suspected and antibiotics considered.

If a doctor sends a white blood cell count on your febrile child, ask how the result will affect his/her care. Often we send a CBC to help make the decision between a "sick" and a "well" child. Certainly you will feel that your vomiting, crying, febrile, child is sick, but the doctor in this instance is trying to determine if the cause of the fever is a routine viral infection, often known as a common cold, or if the cause is something more serious, such as pneumonia, a difficult-to-detect urinary-tract infection, or possibly something even worse, such as meningitis (infection of the brain, fluid, and tissue surrounding it). The white blood count and types of white blood cells provide just one more bit of information, and not the entire answer. An elevated white blood cell count should prompt further testing, treatment, and possibly observation or admission.

Blood Chemistry Testing

The human body is an amazingly stable and resilient system, and unless there is a reason to suspect an abnormality, routine testing of blood chemistries is far more likely to show abnormal values as a result of lab error than as a result of actual imbalances. If you are going along, doing well, and your doctor recommends a routine blood chemistry panel, you should ask, "What are you looking for?"

A basic chemistry panel contains levels of sodium, potassium, chloride, bicarbonate, blood urea nitrogen, creatinine, and glucose. Sodium, potassium, and chloride are the basic intra- and extracellular chemicals. An abnormality of these should be suspected with prolonged vomiting or diarrhea (with or without dehydration), diuretic use, or excess water drinking. Of the three, sodium is unique, as low sodium can cause changes in mental status. Elderly patients and psychiatric patients who suddenly do not know who they are or where they are occasionally are found to have low sodium. A normal sodium level is about 140 (milligrams per deciliter). Changes start at a sodium level of about 125, and by 115, many people don't know where they are or even who they are anymore.

My first experience with hyponatremia (low sodium) was when I was a third-year medical student on my internal medicine rotation in Cleveland. I was in charge of admitting and caring for a ninety-one-year-old woman named Esther. Esther had lost her husband as a result of a fall that caused a hip fracture five months earlier. She was very sad, as they had been married for over sixty years. She was unable to manage at home without her husband and was placed in a nursing home. Esther had worked as a beautician until she was eighty-nine, which I found remarkable, since her hair was a complete mess and she didn't seem to care.

To treat her depression, she was placed on an antidepressant. A common side effect of antidepressants is dry mouth. Without realizing it, and probably because her short-term memory was not as good as it once was, Esther drank a lot of water. During our initial interview, which was about an hour long (medical students do huge write-ups), she asked for water at least four times. Her primary treatment was to be water restriction. Her sodium level was to be rechecked twice per day. Generally the sodium corrects very quickly.

At rounds the next day, I presented the sodium as unchanged at 114! We considered brain tumors, cancers, and other possible causes, and I had prepared an extensive "differential diagnosis list." None of the other things fit, and we had already ruled out most of them. The professor said, "Figure it out, Borden."

Chapter 30 The Medical Laboratory

I started by asking the nurses if Esther was following her fluid restriction. Her day nurse said she had asked for water several times each hour for the first morning, but then had stopped asking. The water to her sink had been turned off because the nurse saw her fill an empty juice container there on the first day.

I parked my chair outside her room with my books in a position where I could see the full-length mirror just inside the door. It didn't take long until she swung out of bed and headed for the bathroom. I peeked around the corner and sure enough, ninety-one-year-old Esther was kneeling down and scooping water out of the toilet! We shut off and dried up the toilet, giving her a bedside commode, and the next morning I was greeted by a very different person. Her sodium had risen to 125 and she said, "Good morning, Doctor Borden!" That was the first time she had used my name. She was in front of the mirror doing her hair!

Potassium can often be depleted by diarrhea or diuretic use. Other things that cause increased urination, such as diabetes and excess fluid consumption, can also cause low potassium. Low potassium is called hypokalemia. *Hypo*kalemia is generally not dangerous (we'll talk about *hyper*kalemia next, which is dangerous), but low potassium does make a person feel weak and "washed out."

Medical people often make the mistake of worrying too much about low potassium levels. In general, compulsively correcting abnormal lab values can be a problem, and when it comes to potassium, this can be deadly. Lots of people who go into medicine tend to be detail oriented, and it is easy to focus on correcting a number. When I was a medical student, we gave a lot of potassium replacement through the IV. This was very painful for the patient, since potassium burns and destroys the vein through which it is given. Adding some lidocaine helps with the pain, but the vein is still damaged. Potassium is easily taken orally, is well absorbed, and should be given that way if at all possible. There is also the danger that the low potassium result may have been a laboratory error, and if given rapidly intravenously, the much more dangerous problem of hyperkalemia could result. Given orally, there is little risk of accidental hyperkalemia, since potassium is absorbed more slowly and a normal kidney can keep up with its elimination. Hence the saying: "The dumbest kidney is still smarter than the smartest intern."

As a professor, I have often had to convince my residents that aggressive potassium replacement is a bad policy. I ask if they have ever heard of a person dying of low potassium. The answer is invariably "no." I then ask if they have ever heard of someone dying of high potassium, and the answer is just as certainly "yes." Next, I remind them of a syndrome called "familial periodic hypokalemic paralysis." FPP is a genetic problem that causes low potassium. Patients complain of intermittent weakness, which generally causes difficulty climbing stairs. When the potassium gets down to levels that are lower than those we ever see in normal people, weakness can become severe. There are some helpful medicines, and these patients lead full lives. I next ask them if they have heard of genetic hyperkalemia. The answer is "no" and that is because it would not be compatible with survival.

The commonest cause of a high potassium (written on the lab slip as K+) is…sure enough, that recurrent demon: lab error. In the case of falsely elevated potassium, the false elevation is often caused by cells broken during the process of drawing the blood. Cells can also break if there is a delay in analysis. Cells have a high concentration of potassium, and if cells are broken, the potassium (checked in the serum, not within the cells) is falsely elevated. Breaking of cells is known as "hemolysis." The lab will often note this, and the slip may say, "hemolysis present." Truly high potassium is most often caused by renal (kidney) failure, or a decrease in renal function. High potassium causes a change in, and then a cessation of, cardiac electrical conduction. No electrical conduction is *no good*! In patients on dialysis, high potassium is always a concern and routinely checked.

Bicarbonate (written HCO3-) is mostly a measure of acidity. A decreased "bicarb" on the chemistry means there is a state of "acidosis" in the body. Acidosis can result from many causes, but is always important to note. A severe acidosis will require hospital admission. Probably, the most common cause of serious acidosis that we see is caused by untreated, or inadequately treated, type one (juvenile-onset) diabetes. This is called "diabetic ketoacidosis." The problem in diabetes is that the diabetic cannot utilize glucose (sugar) normally. Insulin is needed to move the glucose into the cells, where it can be used. If there is not enough insulin, or if the body cannot use insulin, fats are burned instead, resulting in the production of the acid and ketones—hence the "keto" in ketoacidosis. In diabetic ketoacidosis, a bicarbonate level of less than ten is not unusual.

Blood urea nitrogen (BUN) and creatinine are measures of kidney function. An elevated BUN and creatinine signal failure of the kidneys to eliminate these waste products. Temporary elevations can be caused by urinary-tract blockage or dehydration. Interns and medical students learn early on that when a male of middle age or older has an elevated BUN and creatinine, check the bladder. Prostate enlargement and/or infection can cause the bladder to fill with urine, backing pressure to the kidneys and preventing further urine production. If this happens quickly, it is hard to ignore, but if it happens slowly, or if the patient is normally a bit confused, they are often unable to say, "I really have to go!" Older males who become confused and disoriented are often found to be suffering from urinary retention. We'll discuss this in greater detail in the "Urinary Problems" chapter

Glucose level (blood sugar) is the last number in the basic chemistry. Glucose level in the body is controlled by an interaction of several factors. When a person eats, the nutrition is absorbed. and the level of nutrients, of which glucose is one, increases in the blood. The glucose rise causes the pancreas to excrete insulin into the blood. Insulin causes the glucose to go into the cells. When your glucose is tested immediately after eating, it will naturally be a bit higher. A fully functioning pancreas will secrete enough insulin, and the insulin will be used effectively to keep the glucose level from rising too much. If the pancreas becomes less effective, the glucose will increase after eating for a bit, but then be brought back under control. A first glucose check is often done randomly. If a high result occurs, or if there are other reasons to suspect a problem, a more thorough series of tests can be done.

Glucose can be checked with either a "finger stick" or as a part of a blood-draw chemistry panel. The finger stick, often known as an "accu-check," is faster but less accurate. Accu-checks are especially inaccurate at the higher levels. In the ED we often use a finger stick initially if a person comes in (usually is brought in) with an alteration in mental status. Finger sticks are also often used as we correct the blood glucose level in a diabetic patient.

Reasons to suspect high blood-glucose levels (diabetes) include excessive thirst and increased quantity of urine and a family history of diabetes. Pregnancy can sometimes result in a temporary problem with increased blood-glucose levels, and since these high levels can result in large babies and difficult births, as well as problems shortly after birth, blood-sugar testing is routine in pregnancy.

Excessive urination results from glucose levels consistently near or over two hundred milligrams per deciliter. At these levels, the sugar (glucose) escapes into the urine. The kidneys cannot stop additional water from being drawn into the urine to dilute this glucose. Thirst results from this loss of water, and excessive drinking, known as polydipsia, is the result. When a diabetic can no longer drink enough water to keep up, severe dehydration occurs, which, combined with the acidosis we discussed above, can result in death. If the blood sugar has been in the two hundred-plus range (more than twice normal), checking the urine for glucose will detect diabetes.

A thorough evaluation to rule out diabetes will include a fasting glucose level and a test after consuming something. Usually a sweet drink of some sort that contains a known amount of glucose is given, and the blood-glucose level is checked at intervals.

Other chemistry tests are specific to certain organs. There are several blood tests for pancreatitis, for example. To look for pancreatitis (inflammation of the pancreas) blood amylase and lipase levels are checked. Amylase and lipase are involved in the digestion of carbohydrates and fats, respectively, and are normally found in the blood in only small amounts. If the pancreas is inflamed or blocked off, more lipase and amylase escape into the blood.

Similar enzymes that relate to the liver can be checked. When we talked about gallstones in the "Abdominal Pain" chapter, I mentioned the blockage of the gallbladder (bile) duct. If that duct is blocked by a gallstone, the liver enzymes will begin to rise. An enzyme called alkaline phosphatase is more sensitive for this blockage than are the other liver enzymes. A rise in the intracellular liver enzymes, which on your lab sheet will most likely appear as AST and ALT, means damage and inflammation of the liver tissue itself.

When we discussed the causes of jaundice (yellow skin color caused by increased bilirubin), we talked about the bilirubin level. The lab can check this level, then differentiate between a bilirubin increase caused by blockage of the liver's outflow ducts and a bilirubin increase caused by something before the liver has a chance to process the bilirubin. If the cause of the jaundice is hepatitis, the AST and ALT (liver cell enzymes) will be elevated into the thousand-plus range, depending on the stage and severity of the infection. Alcoholic hepatitis is a more gradual attack on the liver, and if a test of the liver enzymes in a person who drinks a lot of alcohol shows them to be elevated, the elevation will normally be in the low hundreds. When the liver is severely damaged—for example in Tylenol overdose— the liver enzymes can be over ten thousand.

Not every person who drinks alcohol will develop liver failure. You have probably heard of cirrhosis of the liver, though. Cirrhosis is the result of scarring that forms a network of fibrous tissue, hardening the liver and preventing normal blood flow. Cirrhosis is not always caused by alcohol and often occurs for no apparent reason. If you or someone you know who drinks has an elevation of the liver enzymes, there is liver damage occurring. In this case an ultrasound or another test of the liver could be used to look for scarring, and if scarring is present, a gastroenterologist or hepatologist (liver specialist) should be consulted.

If alcohol is determined to be the cause, all alcohol consumption must be stopped. As the liver becomes scarred, blood flow through it becomes more difficult, and it begins to lose function. The end result of progressive cirrhosis is liver failure. The liver makes some components of the blood responsible for clotting, and bleeding becomes a problem. Possibly worse is the huge amount of fluid that begins to accumulate in the abdomen (called ascites). The liver is one of those things (like the pancreas) that is best left unmolested. Liver failure caused by alcohol is a lingering and ugly death.

Urinalysis

The urinalysis is an especially useful and easy test since no pain is involved and no radiation required. The urine can give many clues and may lead to other tests to confirm diagnoses that the urine hints at. For instance, if bilirubin is found in the urine, a blood bilirubin level may find an elevation that will result in an important diagnosis.

Chapter 30 The Medical Laboratory

In 1675 Thomas Willis added the word "mellitus," which stems from honey, to the word diabetes when he noticed (as had been noted for centuries) that the urine of a diabetic patient tasted sweet. Analysis of the urine is no longer done by taste luckily!

Two methods are generally employed in analyzing urine. First the urine is tested chemically, usually with a "urine dip." A strip containing a series of colored tabs that react to measure the various properties is dipped in the urine. After the chemical test, and generally if the chemical test shows an abnormality, the urine is examined microscopically (or inserted into a machine that examines it). The two chemical indicators of infection are leukocyte esterase and nitrates. If one or both of these are present, a microscopic examination will be done to look for white blood cells, which indicate infection. Blood in the urine is also detected with the dip and unless it is expected (menses) seeing blood on the dip will also lead to further analysis.

As we discussed earlier in this chapter, the urine can look cloudy, bloody, and even "purulent" (milky, containing pus) in the case of serious infection. Badly infected urine also smells foul, generally, and some infections cause more odor than others.

In general a darker (darker yellow, usually) urine is more concentrated. The "specific gravity" of a urine specimen is measured, both with the urine dip and urinalysis. Specific gravity is usually measured up to a level of 1.030 (pronounced "ten-thirty"). A urine found to have a specific gravity of 1.005 is very dilute, and a urine with a specific gravity of 1.030 is very concentrated. A pregnancy test done early in pregnancy is more accurate if the urine is concentrated.

The urine dip will detect glucose, and therefore a urine dip is a quick and painless test to screen for diabetes. As we mentioned earlier, though, the blood glucose needs to be about twice normal to spill over into the urine, and early/borderline diabetes can thus be missed.

Medical Wisdom

Ketones in the urine indicate that fat is being broken down. Ketones are often present during dieting, and often are found when a person has been nauseated or vomiting with decreased food intake.

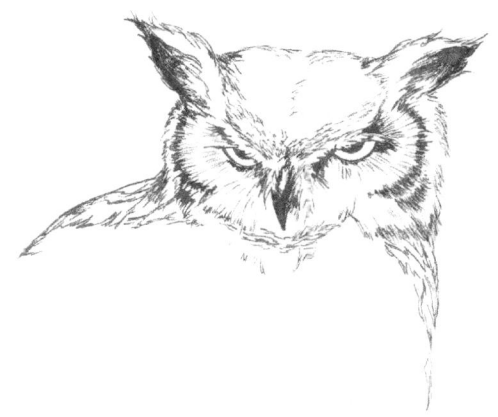

Chapter 31
Medications

One pill makes you larger, and one pill makes you small.

And the ones that mother gives you,

Don't do anything at all.

Go ask Alice,

When she's ten feet tall

—from the song "White Rabbit" by Jefferson Airplane

Certainly medications are to the doctor what a hammer is to the carpenter. I like the saying, "When all you have is a hammer, everything looks like a nail." A lot of things can be fixed with a hammer—but some can be broken in the process!

As a teenager I used a hammer to unstick my truck's starter. I would turn the key and hear only a whirr. After a few whacks with the hammer, it would start right up. It worked again and again until I'd saved up enough money to buy a new starter. To save money, I changed the trucks oil and filter myself (I still do). The oil filter was shaped just like the starter, but when I tried the hammer on the stuck oil filter, things didn't work out as well!

There are a lot of excellent medications that can easily help when given in the right circumstances. Some of these medications are essentially harmless, and if they don't help, they probably won't hurt either. Some medications have real, substantial downsides, though. Whenever your doctor suggests a new medication, be sure to ask about the possible problems that may result.

Drug Interactions

If you are on other medications and your doctor wants to add one, ask if there will be any adverse drug interactions. Also, when you are started on a new medication, ask if that particular medication has problems "getting along" with other medications in general. Some medications are just plain problematic.

The best example of this is the blood-thinning drug Coumadin. Coumadin is a touchy drug used to slow blood clotting when clots are or may be a potential problem. Coumadin is used after some intra-vascular (inside vessels) procedures; when irregular heart rhythms could cause clots in the heart that might break off and flow to the brain, resulting in stroke; and often for blood clots in the legs (deep venous thrombosis) that can break off and go to the lungs (pulmonary embolus). If you are on Coumadin (also known as warfarin), you are familiar with the regular testing required to ensure the blood-clotting speed stays in the right range. Eating foods rich in vitamin K can stop

Chapter 31 Medications

the action of Coumadin, and a person who eats a lot of greens will need a higher dose than a "meat and potatoes" person. A number of medications have the opposite effect, making the blood get too anti-coagulated, which can result in bleeding.

There are many classes of medications, and to discuss them all in this chapter is not feasible. Also, some types of medication are best addressed in other chapters. In the "Infection" chapter, for example, we talked about antibiotics; in the "Abdominal Pain" chapter, we discussed some medications to stop stomach acid; in the "Hypertension" chapter, we discussed medications commonly used for high blood pressure. Associating those particular medications with the maladies that they treat is a better way to remember them. In the "Shortness of Breath" chapter, we will discuss the steroids used in asthma and COPD.

I am often asked if there is a difference between generic medication and name brands. The active ingredient should be the same and present in the same measured quantity. Sometimes there is a definite difference in the quality of the preparation, though. For example, Advil is covered with a polished, sweet coating that makes it easier to swallow than generic ibuprofen. Advil also costs more, so you'll have to try both and see if the difference is worth it to you.

Some ingredients are used to bind the pills together, and certainly it is possible to be allergic to or intolerant of one of those. In that case there may be a difference between the different brands, be they generic or brand name.

In the next chapter, we will discuss an example of a medication that, though highly effective, was too expensive to use in most cases until the patent ran out. Once generics are available, the name brands also come down in price to compete. Pharmaceutical companies know how much more people are willing to pay for the name brand, and if sales decrease, the price of the name brand will decrease to remain competitive.

Allergy or Intolerance?

What about allergies to medications? Some patients have true allergies to certain medications. One of the most notable is the allergy to penicillin. An allergy is the body's reaction to a substance that sets off a series of symptoms. The most typical symptom of an allergy is hives. Hives are suddenly appearing, itchy thickenings of the skin. Hives can involve the skin only or can involve the mouth, tongue, lips, and face. An extension of hives is swelling of the airways—and not just the mouth, but the lungs themselves.

It is very important to differentiate between allergy and intolerance. Sometimes I see a patient with a long list of allergies, but when I question them, they actually have never had hives, swelling, or any of the true manifestations of an allergy. Usually they complain of stomach upset when taking the medicine or of not liking how the medication made them feel. Stomach upset is not an allergy. Many pills are hydrophilic (tend to rapidly absorb water/moisture) and will stick to the stomach wall if the stomach is empty, in the same way that they will stick to the tongue. The stomach rebels in this instance, contracting in a reflexive effort to stop the potential damage the adherent pill may do to the stomach lining. In these cases, taking the medicine with food should help, or using a liquid formulation may be the answer.

Other pills actually cause some increase or decrease in stomach activity as an effect of their action. Note I say an "effect" and not a "side effect." The antibiotic erythromycin is such a medication. Erythromycin speeds stomach contraction and is sometimes used to increase the function of a slow stomach. On the opposite end of the spectrum are codeine and the other opiates, such as Vicodin, Percocet, morphine, and so on. These medications all slow the stomach. If the stomach is slowed, the body says, "Oh no…things slowing down, reject contents!" As a result, all the opiates cause nausea to some degree, whether taken orally or given through an IV. The opiates also cause constipation by reducing the speed/function of the GI tract. For this reason I always give medication to prevent nausea when giving IV opiates, and stool softener when I prescribe oral opiates.

It is vital to distinguish between these intolerances and true allergies to prevent the elimination of valuable medications from those available to you. Intolerances can almost always be managed, if the benefit of the medication makes it worthwhile. Mild allergies can also be managed, if the benefit is worth the hassle. But severe allergic reactions (anaphylaxis) must be avoided.

I recently reviewed a case where a patient was treated with a much more expensive and more problematic antibiotic because of an intolerance that was listed as an allergy. In this case the patient, who was a thirty-three-year-old elementary schoolteacher, came to the ER with pinkeye (conjunctivitis). Erythromycin was listed as an allergy. The physician wanted to use erythromycin ophthalmic ointment, but instead used Gentamycin ointment. Gentamycin, though effective against pinkeye, causes inflammation of the eye in a large number of cases, especially if used for more than a few days. (You may remember that problem from the "Eye Emergencies" chapter.) In this case the eye began to improve, but then became redder, which naturally caused the conscientious teacher to apply the ointment more often. When she came for her second ER visit, the eye was redder and angrier than ever. The second physician asked about the "allergy," which was actually a stomach upset (intolerance) that would most likely not have even occurred with the low dose that the ointment entails. By heeding a misunderstood "allergy" and thus avoiding the benign, inexpensive medicine, an uncomfortable problem resulted.

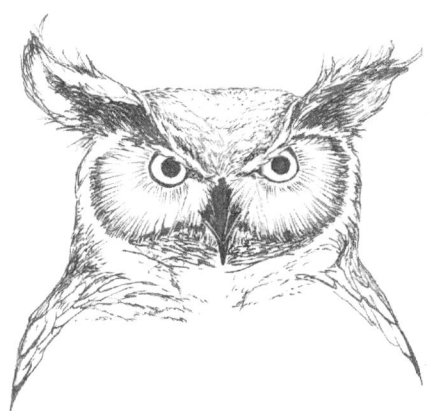

Chapter 32
Nausea, Vomiting, and Diarrhea

There are only two reasons to sit in the back row of an airplane;
either you have diarrhea, or you're anxious to meet people who do.

—Henry Kissinger

In medical school, the professors made a big point—and made it repeatedly—that diarrhea is not watery stool, but a "larger than usual quantity of stool." Since people rarely measure the weight or quantity of their bowel movements, that bit of data has proven of no use whatsoever to me. Most people consider diarrhea to be watery stool, and often recurrent, bothersome watery stool.

Medical Wisdom

There are a lot of causes of nausea, vomiting, and diarrhea. Certainly the commonest is a viral infection of the gastrointestinal tract (commonly referred to as stomach flu). Sometimes these infections are caused by a generalized virus and accompanied by the usual runny nose, sore throat, and cough, but sometimes the symptoms they cause are localized to the GI tract. Luckily, the infections localized to the GI tract are often shorter in duration than the usual viral syndrome. There is not much to do if the stomach flu strikes. Staying well hydrated is good, and drinks such as Gatorade are best, since they replace some of the potassium and sodium lost in diarrhea. If the vomiting is too severe to keep up with the fluid lost, then an antiemetic is needed.

There is now a great antiemetic available known as Zofran. Ten years ago, Zofran (ondansetron) was too expensive for general use and was reserved for cancer patients with the severe, refractory vomiting caused by chemotherapy. Now it is no longer under patent and is affordable. One of the best things about Zofran (ondansetron) is an orally dissolving form that is very effective. Another good thing is that side effects are essentially nonexistent. Zofran is great for use in even small children. Zofran has allowed me to send many children home who years ago would have required intravenous fluids and probably an overnight stay in the hospital.

Fluid is lost from the body by several routes. Imperceptible losses include water vapor from breathing and losses through the skin. Loss of water through the skin becomes noticeable at higher temperatures, but even at a comfortable room temperature, water is continuously lost through the skin. Do you notice that holding someone's hand for a while results in a sweaty palm? That is because the water that is constantly being lost from the skin is held in place by the other person's hand, rather than evaporating into the air. And yes, if the hand was attached to someone special, excitement may have played a part!

Vomiting and diarrhea result in major increases in fluid loss. The lost fluid is not just water, either, but a mix of electrolytes. Vomiting and diarrhea are to a degree "self-limited," since a dehydrated person will naturally vomit less and have less diarrhea than a well-hydrated person. but becoming that dehydrated feels bad and is a major system stress.

Is Dehydration Present?

It's important to be able to judge whether or not dehydration is present. If you are judging your own or another adult's hydration status. consider the answer to the question, "Are you thirsty?" as a place to start. Thirst sometimes lags behind dehydration, but not far behind! Sometimes nausea will kill thirst, though, so looking for a dry mouth can help. Dark, concentrated urine is an indication of dehydration. The kidneys will be hanging onto every bit of water, and thus the urine will contain more waste products and less water per a given volume. "Capillary refill" is often used in both children and adults to judge the state of hydration. We have already discussed this in another context, but it is worth repeating. Choose a place on your palm or nail bed, and with a finger from the other hand press firmly. Notice that when you release the pressure, the area is blanched pale, but then "refills" with blood, assuming a redder color. With normal blood volume (hydration) and circulation, this refilling takes less than two seconds.

Dehydration lowers the circulating blood volume, and with less blood volume, the body's natural response is to decrease the blood flow to the arms and legs (extremities), in an effort to ensure that the vital organs have enough blood. This decrease in blood flow causes the delay of capillary refill. When you feel your child's hands and feet, notice their temperature. Being cold can also delay capillary refill, as blood flow can be decreased to the arms and legs in an effort by the body to retain heat.

Medical Wisdom

How, you may ask, can blood volume decrease when we are not actually losing blood? That is a good question and learning the answer is part of a medical student's education. Fluid in the body is considered to be stored in three "compartments": (1) the intravascular compartment (blood stream), (2) the intracellular compartment (within the cells), and (3) the interstitial compartment (between the cells). These three compartments are very much connected. The body is constructed of permeable membranes. When fluid is given through an IV, it goes straight into the bloodstream (vascular compartment), but within seconds, a portion of the fluid leaves the bloodstream and goes into the body's cells and into the spaces between the cells.

Losing Fluid and Losing Blood

Here is a perfect example of this process in action. A regular patient of my hospital had her blood drawn for a routine health check on March 6. Her hematocrit was 40 percent. On March 9 she came in suddenly at about eleven at night, driven by her husband and covered in blood. She had driven home from a late business meeting, locked her keys in the car, and didn't want to wake him up. She tried to open one of the kitchen windows on her house, and since it was sticky, she "threw her weight against it, and it shattered."

She had several small cuts to her hand, but a large one to her upper arm that hit the brachial artery. Her husband was awakened by her cries and had the presence of mind (and medical wisdom) to fasten a makeshift pressure wrap around her arm, which stopped the bleeding, saving her life. He did this by folding up a sink towel and using the power cord from the blender to tie it in place. He then inserted a big wooden spoon between the cord and the towel, and by twisting the spoon, applied pressure. He had her hold the spoon and blender while he drove her to the hospital. The husband said there was "blood everywhere," but could not quantify the loss.

When she arrived I replaced the makeshift tourniquet with a real one, while holding pressure, and examined the wound. Meanwhile my nurse drew her blood and established an IV line. Her first hematocrit was down to 34, even though the blood was drawn only twelve minutes after the wound had occurred. Think about this for a minute: if the blood had been drawn instantly after the wound had occurred, the hematocrit would have been 40, right? Within twelve minutes of the loss, fluids had shifted from those other two compartments, neither of which contains red blood cells, to help refill the intravascular (bloodstream) compartment. In the process her blood was diluted. At that point, she had not received IV fluid.

Since there was nerve and artery damage, she needed to go to surgery. I called and spoke to the surgeon, and he was coming in. I had the nurse draw her blood again to check the hematocrit level. At that point she had received a liter of IV fluid. Her hematocrit returned at 29 percent and was stable at that level when she went to the operating room an hour later. Several units of packed red blood cells were ready to transfuse when she went to the OR. Adding these packed red cells (cells with little or no plasma) raises the hematocrit. She received two units of blood, and her surgeon said her blood loss was very low while doing the repair. She emerged from surgery with a blood count of 34, where it stayed until she was sent home from the hospital the next day. A unit of blood transfused generally raises the hematocrit by three points or so.

Back to Dehydration

Another thing to check if dehydration is suspected is the heart rate. When the body loses fluid, the amount of circulating blood volume is decreased, and the heart will beat faster to compensate for the fact that there is less blood being pumped with each beat. In a young, healthy person, this increase in heart rate is the first "vital sign change" to occur with blood-volume loss.

Skin "turgor" is also sometimes used to judge hydration. In general, older people have poorer skin turgor than young people, though, so this can be a harder test to use for people. It does work well for horses and mules, though. When my mule first starts a race, I can pinch his loose skin on his neck, creating a wrinkle a half-inch high, and it will immediately spring back to flat again. He never wants to drink during the first ten miles or so, and after twenty miles he usually starts drinking. At that point, which is after about two hours of trotting, his skin wrinkle will stay up for two or three seconds before flattening. Some riders peel back their horse's lip and test for refill of the gums in the same way we discussed above. My mule doesn't much like having his lip peeled back, though, and the taste of human skin on his gums makes him open his mouth and shake his head.

Another useful measure of hydration is frequency of diaper wetting or of urination, as well as volume of urine made. When a patient is very ill, a urinary catheter is often placed, and urine volumes are noted to ensure enough IV fluid is being given. It is safe to say that if your child has fewer wet or lighter-weight, strong-smelling diapers, the urine output is decreased. Foul-smelling diapers of normal volume should make you ask about the possibility of a urinary infection. We will discuss urinary infection again in the "Urinary Problems" chapter.

The final result of continued fluid losses in a child is lethargy, weakness, and a limp appearance. If these signs follow diarrhea and/or vomiting, bringing the child to the ER promptly or calling 911 is the best plan.

A little over a month ago, my seven-year-old son, Drake, said he "wasn't feeling so good" after dinner and proceeded to vomit in the wee hours of the morning. He made an acid-smelling, pinkish pool about a foot and a half big on the carpet by his bed. He also sprayed a number of stuffed animals, got the bed sheets real good, and left a trail toward the bathroom. It smelled bad. He felt better and went back to bed (after my wife, Erin, and I spent about an hour cleaning up), but at breakfast time he still looked pale, and instead of eating he vomited again. I pulled out the Zofran orally dissolving tablets and had him take two milligrams under the tongue. He said it tasted like strawberries. Fifteen minutes later, he joined us for breakfast.

If he were a patient of mine in the ER, I would have kept him to clear fluids, but I figured what the heck, can't try this at work (the opposite of "don't try this at home!"). He seemed really hungry and ate a bunch of scrambled eggs and cereal, as well as toast. He looked great and did not vomit again. He did have some diarrhea, though. Three days later, I caught the virus. I was truly nauseated and stood by the toilet several times, but never actually threw up. The diarrhea was impressive. Cleaning up that vomit was a serious exposure to the virus, I suppose, despite my thorough hand washing.

Diarrhea and vomiting are often accompanied by brief, cramping abdominal pain. If the pain is more severe than expected, or if it lasts longer than the usual intermittent cramping, other causes of abdominal pain should be considered. If you are having persistent pain right now, it is time to read the "Abdominal Pain" chapter.

Diarrhea containing blood is also likely to be more serious than a simple viral cause.

Whether or not you "catch" a case of diarrhea depends on the same factors we discussed in the "Cough" and "Infection" chapters. An example of this principle is salmonella. Most people associate salmonella with uncooked chicken and other meat products. Salmonella results in a truly nasty case of diarrhea. A person can ingest some salmonella bacteria without contracting the disease. The vast majority of bacteria are destroyed by stomach acid, and more yet are defeated by the body's intestinal immune system. Of those that get past the stomach acid and immune defenses, the survivors need to compete with the bacteria that already live in the intestinal tract. Therefore, a person needs to ingest a fairly large dose of salmonella to end up with diarrhea. As we discussed in the "Infection" chapter, the degree of exposure is important in determining whether or not clinically evident infection will result.

The disease known as cholera, which is uncommon in developed countries but still a problem in parts of the world, can cause weeks of severe watery diarrhea. Fortunately, the common stomach flu that we see regularly usually only requires a day or two of antiemetic and increased fluids.

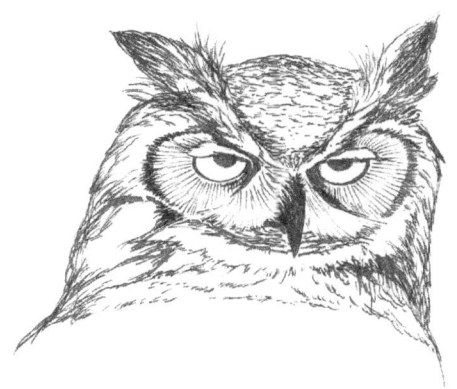

Chapter 33
Pain

Thank you for bringing up such a painful memory. While you're at it, why don't you give a nice paper cut and pour lemon juice in it?

—Miracle Max in the movie *Princess Bride*

Pain is a bit pervasive in the study of medicine, obviously. Almost every chapter in this book discusses pain to some degree, but it is so important that a dedicated chapter is also required to be complete.

Pain is actually of value when it comes to operating the human body successfully. There is a disorder called congenital analgesia, where a person is born unable to feel pain. Sometimes people with this defect can distinguish between hot and cold, but not always. Tongue biting and mouth injury is common, as are eye injuries. Infections are common since the person does not notice an injury or splinter. Fractures are common, and the normal biomechanics are not obeyed. Since a sprained ankle does not hurt, the ankles are injured and wear out quickly. The body becomes a wreck by the time adolescence is reached, if the person survives to adolescence. As you can see, pain is often the body's way of communicating important information.

Pain is often classified into "acute" and "chronic," but it is far from that simple. An acute pain may be a one-time thing, such as with a broken arm, or it may be the acute recurrence of an ongoing problem, such as with kidney stones. Passing a kidney stone is certainly a severe, acute pain, but it will likely recur.

In the ED we treat all sorts of pain, and the options for treatment are many. If the pain is a familiar one to you, then say so and let the physician know why you came in to the ED. Is it worse than usual? Did it resist the usual treatments you use? If the pain is different from the usual pain, such as in the case of a headache, be sure to explain the differences, as such information can affect your treatment greatly.

In recent years a new "vital sign" was added. Most doctors don't like the way it is referred to as a "vital sign" because it is, unlike the real vital signs, subjective. To measure this "vital sign," you will be asked to rate your pain on a one-to-ten scale. Most likely you will be told that "one is a very slight discomfort, and ten is the worst pain you have ever felt." You will then be asked the same question later to see how the treatment is working. The inherent trouble with this scale is that it is not accurate at the high end. Many patients will answer "fifteen" or "way over twenty." The worst pain most people have ever had is the severe pain that is going on right now, which causes all other pains, faded in memory with the passing of time, to seem insignificant by comparison.

Chapter 33 Pain

Most conditions involving recurrent severe pain can be treated initially as needed in the ED, but their ongoing treatment should be by a primary doctor. It is important to have only one source of pain medication prescriptions for a chronic or recurrent painful condition. Many patients have become addicted, overdosed, or otherwise been harmed by receiving prescriptions from multiple doctors. More states are tracking narcotic medication prescriptions in a database. These are then sent to the prescribing physicians if the patient has multiple sources of narcotics. Sometimes receiving these sheets is a real eye opener.

Once I saw a patient for her "first episode of shoulder pain." She fell in the shower, she stated. There was no visible injury and her X-ray was normal, but she was very uncomfortable. I prescribed her fifteen Percocet, our strongest oral narcotic, because she said, "I have tried ibuprofen, and it is not helping. I am allergic to Vicodin." When the tracking sheets arrived, I was surprised to see that I was the fifth doctor she had seen so far that month for pain, at four different ERs! She had been given more than ninety Percocet during the week before coming to see me! I could not imagine her taking all those narcotics herself, and she probably didn't. In some areas Percocet will sell for over ten dollars per tablet on the street. The ER where I currently do most of my clinical work has a very strong policy to decrease narcotic abuse, and every ER needs such a policy.

The first-line medications for pain are generally Tylenol, aspirin, and the other nonsteroidal anti-inflammatory medications, such as ibuprofen. Of these three, most people report the best pain relief with ibuprofen. This may be because it is more effective, or it may be because people know they can take two, three, or even four ibuprofen at a time, while most think only one aspirin can be taken at a time. Of the three, ibuprofen is the least toxic in overdose. A full dose of ibuprofen for an adult should not exceed a hundred milligrams per hour.

Both aspirin and Tylenol cause serious problems in overdose. Aspirin does have some added benefits for people over fifty years of age, since even in small doses, it decreases the risk of heart attack (see the "Chest Pain" chapter) and strokes caused by blood clots (see the "Weakness" chapter). A single eighty-one-milligram aspirin per day is all that is normally recommended for the risk reduction. That small dose is not enough for pain treatment.

Tylenol (acetaminophen) will be discussed in more detail in the next chapter. Tylenol is found in Percocet, Vicodin, and a number of other medications. Since Tylenol (acetaminophen) is toxic in overdose, it is important to know how many total milligrams you are ingesting. I have seen more than a few overdoses that resulted from someone adding Vicodin to the Tylenol they were already taking in an effort to control their pain.

Narcotics definitely have their place in pain treatment. For otherwise healthy people with an acute fracture or other painful injury, they are effective and definitely recommended for the first few days.

Narcotics slow down the gastrointestinal tract; hence, they cause nausea and constipation. Whenever I prescribe narcotics for an older person, I add some stool softener and often an antiemetic. Most shots of narcotic medication in the ED are routinely given with nausea medicine.

Narcotics are both physically and mentally addictive. Some people are not prone to the psychological addiction, but others are. Everyone will become addicted physically, though it takes several weeks or more of continuous use. The degree of physical addiction varies depending on dosage, duration of use, and the individual. Tolerance also becomes a problem, and larger doses are needed as time passes.

In an end-of-life situation, such as with cancer, narcotics are often used for pain relief. In this situation, nausea and constipation are still problems, but tolerance and addiction may be nonissues. If a person has chronic pain from cancer, a combination of continuous narcotics in the form of a patch, supplemented with additional medication as needed, may be the best solution. Then, after several weeks, the patch can be increased if needed to compensate for increased tolerance, and there will be no periods of withdrawal between the oral doses.

When narcotics alone are not enough, they can be combined with other medications. Simply combining with ibuprofen often helps. Adding a benzodiazepine such as Valium (diazepam) or Ativan (lorazepam) can make a big difference. The benzodiazepines, though not pain medications themselves, are synergistic with the narcotics. They also sometimes make people say things like, "Yeah, it still hurts, but I don't care anymore," with a smile. When I was training residents, they would often come to me in frustration after giving a patient multiple doses of morphine without relief. I would go see the patient again with them. First, I would consider the possibility of a nerve block. If the pain was amenable to being treated with a nerve block, we would have complete pain control within minutes, and no more morphine would be needed. No more morphine often meant no more constant nursing attendance (no more risk that the person might stop breathing!) and no more monitoring, which is good for everyone in a busy ED. If a nerve block was not practical—for example, in the case of abdominal pain—adding some Ativan (a benzodiazepine) to the morphine would usually be remarkably effective and a lesson the young doctor would never forget.

For many conditions there are specific pain treatments that are very effective and sometimes curative as well. In the "Headache" chapter, we talked about "temporal arteritis," an inflammation of the temporal artery that causes pain in the area of the temple and headache. Untreated it can lead to blindness. If it is only treated with pain medication, it might feel better, but it will still cause damage, and the chance of blindness is not decreased. Corticosteroids, on the other hand, will cure the condition and stop the pain by stopping inflammation.

A number of new medications are being tried for chronic pain. If you have an ongoing painful problem, you should first seek a diagnosis and treatment. If it eventually appears that an effective treatment is not available and that the pain is going to persist, seeing a pain specialist may be the next step.

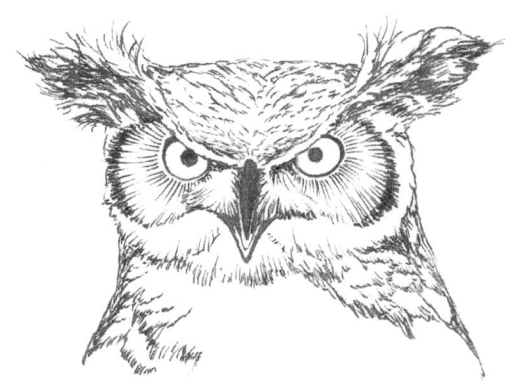

Chapter 34
Pediatric Problems

*There comes a time, thief, when the jewels cease to sparkle, when
the gold loses its luster, when the throne room becomes a prison,
and all that is left is a father's love for his child.*

—King Osiric speaks to Conan in the movie Conan the Barbarian

*We've begun to long for the pitter-patter of little feet—so we
bought a dog. Well, it's cheaper and you get more feet.*

—Rita Rudner

We have been discussing pediatric cases and problems in many chapters, but there are some special considerations worth mentioning.

Medical Wisdom

Any time a child of less than three months of age gets a fever, red flags should wave and warning lights should flash. When I was in medical school and internship, every child less than three months of age with a fever was admitted to the hospital overnight, and all were started on intravenous antibiotic treatment. It was felt that there was such a high risk of serious, life-threatening infection in this age group, that every child needed the maximum antibacterial treatment possible. Since that time, the age limit has relaxed somewhat. New vaccines, such as the haemophilis influenza B vaccine (HIB), have reduced the prevalence of some of the worst pathogens, but still, any fever over 101.5 Fahrenheit in a child less than two months of age is taken very seriously, and most are admitted to the hospital.

Although, after reading the above paragraph, you know my official advice is to take very seriously a fever in a child younger than three months, I should probably tell a brief story to put things in perspective. This story should not change what you do when your child of less than three months has a fever, but it should give you additional information.

When my own son Drake had his first fever, he was only three weeks old. His brother, sister, and mother had all caught a "cold" and all had congestion, fever, and cough. Poor little Drake had the same symptoms. I knew that if I brought him to the pediatrician, he would have blood drawn for labs and culture, an X-ray, a urine catheterization, and a lumbar puncture (spinal tap). I knew, with certainty, that I would also be very strongly encouraged to bring him straight to the hospital for admission and observation. I knew that little Drake had the same viral illness that the rest of my family had and that everything the well-intending doctors and nurses did would be not only useless, but painful to the little guy. I also knew that a stay in the hospital is a great chance for a very young baby to be exposed to some potentially serious infectious problems. I made the choice to keep him at home and treat him the same as our three-year-old daughter. Of course he recovered normally and did just fine.

I absolutely cannot advise you to do the same if your three-week-old gets a fever, but I can advise you to discuss your infant's history and symptoms with the pediatrician in detail before embarking upon an extensive workup to discover the cause of the fever. If a sibling has the same symptoms, and especially if the mother has the same symptoms, be sure to mention it. The sibling and mother are very unlikely to have a serious bacterial disease, and if they have the same problem as the infant, then the infant very probably does not have a serious bacterial disease, either.

Most children will develop a significant diarrhea at some point in their first five years, and this is often rotavirus. The vomiting in rotavirus is usually not severe, but the diarrhea can cause severe dehydration. My own eldest son went from a skinny thirty-one pounds to an emaciated-looking twenty-seven pounds with rotavirus infection when he was two years old. We managed to keep him fairly well hydrated by supplementing his diet with Gatorade and Pedialyte but it was heartbreaking to see him so thin.

Rotavirus can last for up to two weeks, but the worst should be over after the first week. Call the pediatrician for advice; if, despite your efforts, dehydration appears to be occurring, your pediatrician may recommend a trip to the office or ER. Generally, a child with rotavirus will continue to be thirsty, and it is important to give frequent fluids. Small amounts at a time, rather than large amounts, may prevent the vomiting that is triggered by sudden distension of an inflamed stomach. More than two hundred thousand ER visits each year result from rotavirus infection.

Antinausea medication is rarely recommended for children under two years of age, but it can be helpful in older children. Antidiarrheal medication, though commonly used in adults, is also not often recommended in children. Diarrhea is not a disease in and of itself, but a symptom of another problem. Persistent diarrhea (more than two to three days), accompanied by blood or abdominal pain that persists beyond the period immediately preceding the diarrhea, should be a cause of concern.

Small body size can lead to rapid dehydration, rapid cooling if exposed, and faster-than-usual weight loss if food/milk is not tolerated. Children can heal very quickly. I am often amazed at how well a child will recover. Unfortunately, children can also go downhill very fast.

We see a lot of children in the ER. Even so, a call to the pediatrician is a very good idea. Many parents who bring their children into the ER have not called their pediatrician. Even if you are able to reach the advice nurse, rather than the doctor, the call is well worthwhile. A pediatric nurse is an expert at sorting the serious situations from the routine. Routine cases can often wait until the pediatrician is available. Those children with symptoms that may indicate more serious problems should be seen by the pediatrician immediately or go to the ER.

It is amazing and gratifying how well children respond to routine medicines such as ibuprofen (Motrin, Advil). A two-year-old can go from miserable to completely well appearing within ten minutes.

Ibuprofen and Tylenol will also decrease the fever. If the child does look "all better" after the Motrin, it is reassuring. Most serious illnesses will not experience such complete relief. An examination to find the source of the fever, check hydration status, and determine if a problem requiring antibiotics is present will still be required.

Ibuprofen and Tylenol

Ibuprofen and Tylenol (acetaminophen) are worth discussing. Generally, Tylenol is most useful in three instances: In children less than a year old, it may actually work better than ibuprofen. In pregnant women, Tylenol is probably the most benign painkiller. And, because Tylenol is easier on the stomach and esophagus, it is good for patients with gastroesophageal pain, such as gastritis/ulcer.

An important consideration is the comparative potential toxicity of ibuprofen and Tylenol. Most people are not aware that Tylenol accounts for almost five hundred deaths from overdose in the United States each year. An overdose of sufficient size (about ten times the normal dose) is potentially fatal. There are no symptoms of overdose until it is too late. I cared for several Tylenol overdose patients in the ICU as a resident, and the death is slow and far from painless. There is an antidote, which if given early will save the patient. The only "treatment" in the final stages is liver transplant.

Motrin (ibuprofen) on the other hand, can be taken in larger than recommended quantities with no ill effect, or possibly only stomach upset. This difference is important when it comes to children. If a child finds a full bottle of (candy sweet) Tylenol and drinks the whole thing, it is a big problem. If a child finds a full bottle of (candy sweet) ibuprofen and drinks it, there should be no noticeable effect. I recommend all the Tylenol be hunted down and removed from the house when your first child hits one year of age.

There is no doubt that decreasing the availability of Tylenol (acetaminophen) would save at least several hundred lives per year in our country, and I predict that limiting acetaminophen availability and decreasing the doses in acetaminophen-containing medications will be easily accomplished and effective. Just switching from pill bottles to bubble packs might be enough to save several hundred lives each year.

Adults sometimes don't realize that many medications are made with Tylenol as an ingredient. Vicodin and Percocet are two examples. Though these are narcotic pain medications, when a patient arrives with an overdose, it is the Tylenol that is generally the biggest concern, rather than the narcotic.

Urinary-tract infections in children can present differently than in adults. In the very young child, fever and inconsolability may be the only symptoms. A smelly diaper may be a clue. The slightly older child may cry with urination, or hold the urine and not want to go to the bathroom. A child who already mastered use of the bathroom may wet the bed.

Developmental and hormonal problems will usually be picked up by the pediatrician during normal well-child care.

Back to the "Vacs"

It is wise to carefully consider anything that will be injected. Injections bypass the body's normal ability to "avoid things it does not want internalized" and as such merit careful analysis. Injections are uncomfortable and cause kids to cry. Thus vaccines are easy to say "no" to. Vaccination and the associated office visits are also costly. A few weeks ago, my friend Andrew and I were on a long road trip, and the topic of vaccination came up. We calculated the cost of vaccinating his six children and arrived at well over five thousand dollars!

Don't feel you are doing your child a favor by avoiding vaccination, though, because you are not! Just during the approximately twenty years I have been practicing medicine, I have seen major benefit from vaccination. There has been more than a 95 percent reduction in meningitis and epiglottitis from haemophilis influenza type B (HIB) since the vaccine was initiated.

I remember being a hero during my residency when, as a senior, I was called to the operating room by the anesthesiologist to help with a difficult airway in a sick four-year-old boy. The child had epiglottitis. He had been admitted to the pediatric floor from the ER several days before. At that time he could still breathe. Epiglottitis causes severe swelling of the airway, with respiratory distress. Despite antibiotics he had continued to worsen and could barely breathe. The anesthesiologist looked at the airway and knew that since the opening was only a few millimeters and the child was already low on oxygen, it would be a "one-shot deal." We had special equipment for difficult airways in the ER, which we keep in a special box. We kept an intubating stylet in the kit. The intubating stylet fits within the endotracheal tube and can be passed into the narrowed airway, and the tube then eased over it. I used the stylet, and even the narrow stylet was a tight fit into the severely swollen airway. I did pass the tube, over the stylet, and the child ventilated well, with immediate improvement in oxygenation.

I saw quite a few cases of life-threatening epiglottitis and meningitis caused by haemophilis, but now, thanks to the vaccine, the disease that made me a hero, and which killed many children by gradually choking them to death, is so rare that it is essentially never seen (in children). Epiglottitis is now a rare disease of adults who were born before the vaccine! If you still need convincing, go to the CDC (Centers for Disease Control) website and read the section titled "What Would Happen if We Stopped Vaccinations?"

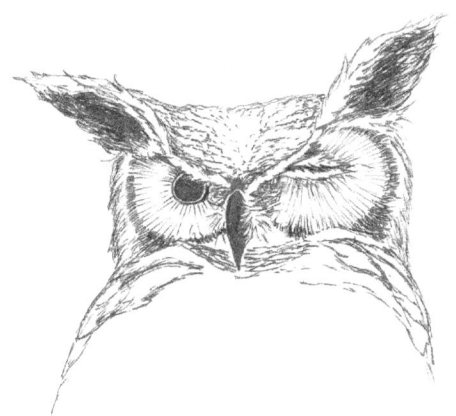

Chapter 35
Penile and Testicular Problems

For most of my life I had operated under a simple schematic of winning and losing, but cancer was teaching me a tolerance for ambiguities.

—Lance Armstrong

The penis is a relatively simple body part and not prone to many troubles. There are a few congenital defects that are often noticed and cared for early, and after that, the problems are limited.

Occasionally in uncircumcised males, the foreskin can cause difficulties. "Phimosis" is the failure of the foreskin to retract. It is normal for the foreskin to not retract in young males, and this is called "physiologic phimosis." As males grow, the foreskin loosens from the head of the penis, largely as a result of intermittent foreskin retraction and erections. Poor hygiene and episodes of infection beneath the foreskin can lead to scarring and inability of the foreskin to retract. If a scarred and tightened foreskin retracts and remains retracted, the foreskin can act as a partial tourniquet. The head of the penis can swell (slowed venous return with continued arterial perfusion), and the resulting problem is called paraphimosis. The head of the penis can get quite large, and it is painful. To reduce a paraphimosis in the ER, I first anesthetize the penis with a nerve block. Then I wrap the head of the penis with a small elastic bandage, forcing some of the blood from the head of the penis back down the shaft. The foreskin can then be replaced and wrapped in place until the remainder of the swelling resolves.

"Priapism" is the persistence of an erection for more than four hours and continuing without sexual purpose or desire. This is a serious problem and not worth explaining here, but needs immediate emergency attention.

Burning of the penile urethra with urination can occur when the urine is concentrated (dehydration) or when there is an infection or injury. The sexually transmitted disease gonorrhea causes severe burning, whereas the disease chlamydia causes milder symptoms usually described as itching. Both of these are treated with antibiotics, and any sexual partners need to be found and advised. Nonspecific urethritis is similar to chlamydia in that it is more irritating than painful. The same antibiotics that work for chlamydia are effective in nonspecific urethritis.

Mild and irritating testicular pain is common and may be positional or occur for no particular reason. Severe pain to one testicle can be serious. Testicular torsion is a very painful problem that occurs when a testicle rotates within the scrotum, kinking the blood vessels and cutting off the blood supply. This problem occurs most frequently in young males. This is an emergency, and if it occurs you should come (or bring your boy) straight to the emergency department.

Chapter 35 Penile and Testicular Problems

The pain of testicular torsion usually occurs suddenly and is severe. It often radiates to the lower abdomen. If your teenager suddenly complains of severe pain of the lower abdomen and appears distressed, testicular torsion is worth considering, as many shy teenagers will hesitate to say "testicle." In the ED an ultrasound will likely be used to check blood flow to the testicles. If it is found to be decreased, the testicle can possibly be "detorsed" (untwisted) by hand. Looked at from the front, the direction to rotate the testicle is away from the midline, as if opening a book. Immediate pain relief should occur if the detorsion is a success. Some 65 percent of testicular torsion occurs in boys between twelve and eighteen years of age.

Infection of the testicle—the epididymis—results in pain and swelling. Epididymitis is the commonest cause of testicular pain and swelling. The epididymis is a thickened structure on the testicle where sperm matures after leaving the testicle and entering the vas deferens (tube that leads away from the testicle). One of my favorite jokes is to ask a person who has done something especially brilliant if anyone has ever "called you an epididymis?" They always say, "Well, no," or some such, to which I reply, "You know—on the ball!"

In epididymitis, the entire testicle feels swollen and tender; however, an ultrasound will show that the testicle is of normal size, but that there is a fluid collection around it that is making it feel and look bigger. Antibiotics are the treatment, with urology follow up. The same bacteria that cause sexually transmitted diseases and urinary-tract infections are generally the cause.

Orchitis is the inflammation of the testicle itself. Orchitis is less common, especially now that mumps (which was a typical cause) has been nearly eliminated by vaccination. Epididymitis can spread to the testicle. The treatment is similar, and urologic consultation may be required.

Self-examination of the testicles is important. Monthly exams are recommended and only take a few seconds. Anything that feels new or out of place should prompt an immediate trip to the doctor. Testicular cancer, like breast cancer, is usually very treatable if caught early.

Male impotence is a fairly common problem with a large number of diagnosable causes. Reportedly, only a small percentage of men with impotence seek treatment. Several new drugs are now available that have many previously hopeless cases "popping up" to take a look. Viagra, is the first reliably effective oral agent for impotence. It should not be used with nitrates, however, and there are some other side effects to discuss with your doctor before taking it.

Viagra does not magically cause an erection, but can facilitate an erection when combined with the right mental and physical cues. The first time I prescribed Viagra for a friend he reported a complete failure. He is a firefighter and decided to try it after a hard day at work. He got home, opened a beer, sat down on the couch and swallowed a Viagra. Several hours went by while he watched TV, and "nothing happened at all." He expected that an erection, and possibly a bigger one than usual, would just occur as the pill "kicked in." I asked him what he watched on TV. He replied; "just football highlights and stuff." I reassured him that he had experienced a normal reaction, and should not give up hope just yet.

In medical school we were taught that there are two main categories of impotence: psychological and physical. We were told that if normal nocturnal erections occur, then the cause is psychological. Nocturnal erections are known as "nocturnal penile tumescence"; their cause is not known with complete certainty, but it is thought they are the result of the relaxation of inhibitory neurons during REM (rapid eye movement) sleep. A device can be worn on the penis at night to record these tumescent periods, and that may be the first step in the diagnosis of impotence.

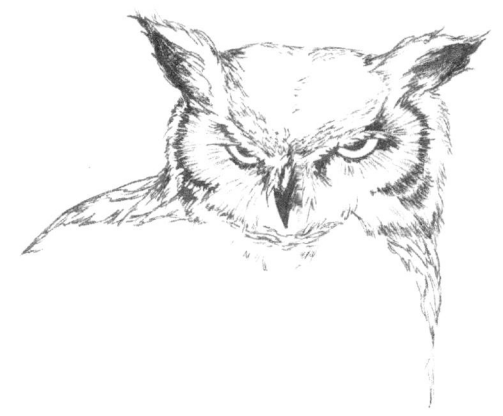

Chapter 36
Pregnancy-related Problems

It is now quite lawful for a Catholic woman to avoid pregnancy by resorting to mathematics, though she is still forbidden to resort to physics or chemistry.

—H. L. Mencken

Many problems are unique to pregnancy, and though this chapter will be a good overview, if you are pregnant, you will benefit from another text as well. I recommend *What to Expect When You're Expecting* by Heidi Murkoff. Also, there is no substitute for good prenatal care.

Pregnancy is broken down into three sections. These are called the first, second, and third trimesters. Problems are different as the pregnancy progresses. We will start with the first trimester.

271

First Trimester Problems

In the first trimester, the commonest problems that cause visits to the ER are pelvic pain, vaginal bleeding, and nausea with vomiting. Morning sickness can be the first sign of pregnancy. Generally this nausea is limited to the first trimester, but it can sometimes last longer. Many women find some relief by eating dry toast, crackers, and other bland food. If that fails, there are a number of antiemetics that work well. We talked about some good ones in earlier chapters, including the "Nausea, Vomiting, and Diarrhea" chapter.

If you have a lot of nausea and vomiting, treatment is important for several reasons. Dehydration can contribute to urinary-tract infections, which are harder to notice in pregnancy and can increase the chance of miscarriage. During the first three months, the baby is not growing much as far as poundage is concerned, but he or she is becoming fully formed, and malnutrition or other bad habits, such as alcohol use/drugs/smoking, can cause serious problems. Severe vomiting can decrease a woman's overall nutrition and health, and that is not good during this critical period. Though it is best to minimize medication use during pregnancy, the antinausea medicines are generally OK. Most obstetricians have their favorite antiemetic, and asking yours for their suggestion is wise.

Planning for pregnancy is best because prenatal vitamins taken early are most beneficial, and often a woman will not be able to tell that she is pregnant for the first month or even two. The first month is an important time to avoid medication, drug and alcohol use, and smoking. With a planned pregnancy, a healthier first few months can be thoughtfully arranged.

Miscarriage is mostly a first-trimester problem. Many pregnancies are lost before the woman even knows she is pregnant. In many cases this is actually a good thing, as something abnormal has probably occurred, whether it is an inadequate placenta or error in development. Miscarriage is not an easy thing to go through. There is no way to make it easy. The good news is that as the pregnancy proceeds, miscarriage becomes less likely. Less than one woman in a hundred will miscarry after the first trimester.

The terms abortion and miscarriage are often used interchangeably in the medical world, even though to the layman, abortion is very different from miscarriage.

There is a stressful condition in which the fetus is found to be nonviable (either no longer growing or deceased) and yet a miscarriage is not happening. This is referred to as an "inevitable abortion." In the case of an inevitable abortion, D and C (dilatation and curettage) can be done to end the pregnancy. If time is allowed to pass, though, things will generally progress naturally. D and C is not painless, often includes the risks of anesthesia, and is not without complications. Nowadays it should be called a dilatation and suction, rather than a dilatation and curettage, since suction is generally used.

Some women I have diagnosed with a failed pregnancy/inevitable abortion in the ED have returned within a day or two asking for a D and C. In these cases I always advise that the natural course of events is the best, if possible. I stress that D and C is not an immediate "cure" either, and that bleeding usually continues afterward. Scarring of the uterus can occur, as can perforation of the uterus. Sometimes D and C is done for persistent bleeding during a miscarriage, and for that problem it is generally effective.

If you do have bleeding during pregnancy it is important to know your blood Rh type. Since you have read the previous chapters, you will be familiar with the antigen/antibody interaction and the immune system. Rh is an antigen that is present in some people and not in others. If you are pregnant and do not have Rh (i.e., you are Rh negative) and if your baby does, your body could see your baby as something that doesn't belong. There will be no problem as long as there is no crossover of blood between the mother and child. If there is bleeding, there is a good chance that there is some crossover. If the mother is Rh negative, the antibody known as Rhogam can be given. Rhogam will bind to the baby's antigen that has crossed into the mother, neutralizing it before the mother's body can mount an immune response. If Rhogam is not given, succeeding pregnancies with an Rh positive fetus become more difficult. Even if there has not been bleeding during the pregnancy, there is some blood exposure at birth, and Rhogam is given during the last trimester and around the time of birth, if the mother is Rh negative, to prevent sensitization.

In general, if a pregnancy is healthy and normal, no amount of jumping rope, jogging, having sex, or coughing in the first trimester will cause a problem. Conversely, if an early pregnancy is abnormal and bound for miscarriage, there is usually nothing that can be done to save it. Therefore, a woman should not blame herself.

Pain during the first trimester should not be ignored. There will likely be some mild discomfort, but real pain can be the sign of a serious problem. An ectopic, or "tubal," pregnancy is a possibility in the first trimester. In most parts of the United States, an ultrasound will be done at some point to determine the due date and to look for any problems. At this time the location of the baby and placenta will be noted. If the baby is found to be in the uterus, all is generally well. An ectopic (outside of the uterus) twin is possible but very rare.

In an ectopic pregnancy, the fertilized egg either doesn't make it into the fallopian tube (which leads to the uterus), or it implants in the tube. The tube can support an early pregnancy, but development will not proceed normally, and pain, rupture of the tube, and possibly bleeding of such severity as to be a danger to the mother can occur. An ectopic pregnancy should be suspected if there is unusual pain and bleeding early in the pregnancy. If you have bleeding and pain in the first trimester, an ultrasound will be done to rule out ectopic pregnancy.

Of course the usual problems, such as appendicitis, can occur during pregnancy. Doctors' natural tendency is to focus on pregnancy-related problems when they hear of abdominal pain in pregnancy, but it is important to remember the usual suspects.

Chapter 36 Pregnancy-related Problems

Gallbladder-related pain, which we discussed in detail in the "Abdominal Pain" chapter, can be a frequent problem in pregnancy, but in general, surgery is avoided during pregnancy if possible.

Appendicitis can be a bit trickier during pregnancy because as the uterus enlarges, the appendix moves up in the abdomen and begins to imitate the right-upper-quadrant pain of the gallbladder. This is not much of a problem in the first trimester, but it becomes more notable as the uterus enlarges. Since gallbladder pain is common in pregnancy, it is fairly easy for a doctor to forget about the "relocated appendix," instead focusing on the gallbladder.

Sexually transmitted diseases can still be contracted during pregnancy and are generally screened for to ensure they are treated or the infant is guarded during birth. Even with screening, it is still standard to apply erythromycin ointment to the eyes of each newborn baby to treat possible exposure to chlamydia during birth.

Second Trimester

The second trimester is usually smoother. The nausea and risk of loss are mostly left behind. There is an occasional bit of remnant nausea, usually toward the first few weeks.

Cervical incompetence, if it is going to be a problem, will usually become an issue in the second trimester. The cervix is the muscular opening of the uterus, and usually it remains closed until labor. If the cervix begins to loosen and open ahead of time, an early delivery or miscarriage can result. Sometimes a strong suture known as a "cerclage" can be used to help the cervix remain closed. Bed rest is often needed if this is a problem.

The cervix is usually long and thick. What is meant by "long" is best pictured by visualizing the uterus as a bottle with a neck, like a wine bottle. The cervix is the neck of the bottle. If the baby is in the bottle, and the baby begins to apply force toward the neck of the bottle, the neck of the bottle can begin to "shorten," going from a neck like a wine bottle toward one like a milk bottle, and then, when the cervix shortens enough, it has no choice but to begin to open. Ultrasound can examine the cervix to see if it is shortening, or thinning, and the cerclage can be placed if needed.

Third Trimester Problems

In the third trimester, the mere size of the pregnancy causes discomfort. It is also normal to have some contractions. These are usually weak, compared with the contractions during labor, and are irregular. These early contractions are called "Braxton Hicks contractions." If the contractions become painful, regular, and closer together, you might be going into labor.

Some shortness of breath during pregnancy is not unusual. This is mostly due to the pressure of the baby on the diaphragm, which separates the chest from the abdomen. A woman in the third trimester is also carrying a lot of extra weight, which makes normal daily activity more difficult. If you feel the shortness of breath is suddenly worse or different than expected with abdominal fullness, you should call your doctor. We will discuss shortness of breath in great detail in its own chapter.

Backaches, frequent urination, leg swelling, varicose veins, and hemorrhoids are some other unpleasant things typical of the last part of pregnancy. If you have experienced pregnancy, then enough said. If you have not…then enough said!

Bleeding in the third trimester can be caused by several serious problems. A small amount of bleeding is normal as the cervix dilates shortly before and during labor. A large amount of blood without labor or with pain can be one of two serious problems.

"Placenta previa," in which the placenta is located so it covers the cervix, obstructing the baby's exit, is a potentially life-threatening problem. This is detectable with ultrasound, but if no ultrasound is done, it may be missed. The bleeding is bright red, painless, and can be very heavy. C-section is required for delivery and will be scheduled if your ultrasound shows placenta previa.

"Placental abruption" is another cause of bleeding. In placental abruption, the placenta becomes partially detached from the uterus. This can occur spontaneously or as a result of trauma. Ultrasound can differentiate this from a placenta previa. Both the baby and mother are at risk. The baby is at risk because when the placenta is partially detached, the oxygen and nutrient delivery to the baby is decreased. Large volume blood loss can endanger the mother, as well. In placental abruption, hospital admission with fetal and maternal monitoring is required. A decision may be made to deliver by C-section if needed.

The baby's size can be accurately monitored with ultrasound during pregnancy, and you will be told if he or she is too small or large. If you and your siblings were small at birth, and if your husband or wife was also small at birth, then there is a definite tendency toward small babies. If you and your husband were big babies, then big babies are expected.

A few factors can be treated if the baby is found to be either bigger or smaller than predicted. Many women have a temporary tendency toward diabetes during pregnancy. Having higher-than-usual glucose levels can result in a larger-than-expected baby, which may be hard to deliver. A glucose-tolerance test is standard in pregnancy to help ensure a diabetic problem does not exist.

Anemia, malnutrition, placental problems, and a number of other things can cause a smaller-than-expected baby. If your ultrasound or measurements show this to be the case, discuss it in detail with your obstetrician.

Anesthesia during delivery can vary from nothing to general anesthesia. I often hear women talking about their labor experience, and I have personally delivered hundreds of babies. I can state with confidence that delivery ranges from quick and relatively painless, to very long, very painful, and then…to impossible!

The appropriate anesthesia is therefore highly variable and usually requires changes as the labor progresses. Some highly effective nerve blocks can anesthetize the vaginal area, and an epidural or spinal anesthesia are options that allow a woman to remain awake and fully alert, while experiencing less pain. Nerve blocks such as the pudendal block numb the vaginal area, but you will still be able to feel and move your legs. Contractions will still be felt. The epidural takes a bit longer than a spinal to take effect and provides a lower degree of numbing, while still relieving pain.

If the labor is intended to be without any pain control, but then becomes unexpectedly painful, the epidural and spinal anesthetic routes may not be an option, since they take a bit of time to be done and are delayed in their effect.

After a woman's first delivery, she will have a better idea of what to expect. Discussing the options with your OB and also with your anesthetist or anesthesiologist ahead of time is the best plan for your first delivery.

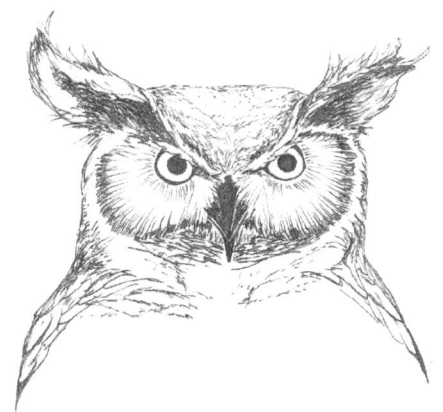

Chapter 37
Psychiatric Problems, Depression, and Suicide

Suicide is a permanent solution to a temporary problem.

—Phil Donahue

While in the ED, expect to hear and see some loud, disruptive, and possibly dangerous patients. Most EDs serve the entire population, and part of our job is to "medically clear" patients for incarceration. Before an injured or intoxicated patient is jailed, they are brought to the ED for evaluation and treatment as needed.

Sometimes the patient potentially is, has been, or just plain is violent and dangerous. I have seen more than a few of my nurses and fellow doctors injured and have been assaulted several times myself. Sometimes the police will remain in attendance for the entire visit, but at other times, they will restrain the patient and be present intermittently. Small-town EDs have a limited police presence, whereas big-city EDs often have full-time officers and lots of available backup. At the university, there was quite a bit of violence, and tranquilizers, restraints, and Taser guns were used regularly. Where gang violence is prevalent, the waiting room itself can become dangerous, as rival gangs assemble to wait while their fellow members are being treated.

Some patients with psychiatric disorders, notably acute psychosis, can become violent and require sedation and restraint. Sedation and restraint are used both to prevent harm to others, and to prevent the patient from self-harm.

When a patient is brought to the ER after having attempted suicide or having spoken about thoughts or a plan to harm him- or herself, the danger is taken very seriously. My primary job as emergency physician is to acquire an understanding of the history of the situation, perform an examination, and then treat the person to stabilize them, preventing physical harm. There is almost always a special consultant, whether it is a social worker or a designated mental health professional who will take a much more detailed history, help me determine the degree of suicidal risk, and arrange psychiatric hospitalization if needed.

Once a patient is determined to pose a suicide risk, the decision is made between voluntary treatment and involuntary treatment facilities. The patient cannot refuse treatment at this point, as he or she is placed on "hold." If needed, the patient can be restrained or guarded by police to prevent self-harm or "elopement."

Chapter 37 Psychiatric Problems, Depression,

A number of things contribute to a risk of suicide. A strong intent and definite plan are two often listed first, and depression and hopelessness are a strong third. An example of someone who doesn't have a definite plan is a young lady I saw three weeks ago. When I asked, "Have you thought about how you will commit suicide?" she replied, "I guess I'll take some pills or something." I asked if she had pills around, or if she had a particular type of pill in mind, and she replied that she had neither pills available nor a particular kind in mind. She was heading toward a low-risk category, thankfully. During the same shift, police brought in a man who had been seen standing on the edge of a high bridge. When I asked him the same question, he replied, "I am going to go back to the bridge, and this time they won't stop me." As you can guess, he was considered at high risk and was hospitalized.

Men are at higher risk of completing suicide than women, and this is mostly because they often choose more violent methods. Women, however, attempt suicide more frequently. Each year, four to five times more males than females commit suicide; surprisingly, females make three times as many suicide attempts as males. Being male is therefore an important risk factor for death by suicide. Suicide risk increases steeply at fourteen years of age, levels off from ages twenty-five to fifty-five, and then increases again to reach the highest rate—about twenty-five per hundred thousand—between seventy-five and eighty-four years of age.

Other factors that clearly increase the risk of suicide are mental illness, substance abuse, and a family history of suicide.

I mentioned above that depression and hopelessness are risk factors for suicide. Clearly if you are dealing with a male relative who is depressed and feeling hopelessness, it is time to call someone for help, or come to the ER. It will be tough to make the judgment call, but certainly it is better to err toward seeking help.

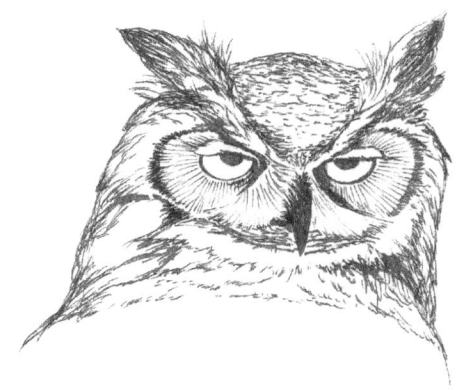

Chapter 38
Shortness of Breath

To many men…the miasma of peace seems more suffocating than the bracing air of war.

—**George Steiner**

What do I mean by "short of breath?" Let's start with what I *don't* mean. I don't mean a stuffed-up, congested nose. A stuffed-up nose is irritating, no doubt, but if it truly becomes totally plugged, breathing through the mouth always remains an option. I suppose if you are kidnapped, your hands tied, and duct tape plastered over your mouth…

I also don't mean the feeling that people often describe as, "I just can't quite take a really deep breath." This is an interesting feeling, sometimes described as the "inability to yawn." If it is pain that is stopping the really deep breath, there are a number of things to consider, but this is not what I mean when I say shortness of breath.

By shortness of breath, medical people mean the feeling of "air hunger." If you run really fast for a while, you will feel this sort of shortness of breath. This feeling results in an increased respiratory rate and often an increased depth of the breaths as well. If you are running fast, your body has an increased need for oxygen and an increased need to eliminate carbon dioxide. These needs result in an increased amount of air that needs to be moved in and out of the lungs per minute (minute volume). Now, imagine yourself with that feeling of needing more air, but you are not running. There is no way to slow down to rest, and even though you are breathing hard and fast, you just can't seem to get enough air. This is shortness of breath. If your palms are not feeling like they are about to sweat, and if you are not a little bit anxious, I have not done an adequate job of explaining the feeling.

What is that Owl Wearing?

Chances are that your doctor will either be wearing a stethoscope around his or her neck, or have one folded in the pocket of their white coat. The stethoscope is mainly used to listen to the sounds of the heart and lungs.

If you do not own a stethoscope, your ear pressed against the chest wall will work just as well. As with the stethoscope, a good seal of the ear (diaphragm or bell in the case of the stethoscope) against the chest is needed. Clothing seems to interfere more when the ear is used directly, than when the stethoscope is used.

When listening to the heart I expect to hear the normal "lub-dub" of the heart and little else. Usually there is a faint sound of blood flow, and that is normal. A louder than normal extra sound is not normal and can indicate a variety of flow problems. When damaged or scarred/malformed the valves cause a heart "murmur." A defect in the dividing wall (septum) between the left and right heart also will cause a murmur. Changes in flow as the heart is stressed will cause an abnormal sound. Some people are born with a murmur, and this may or may not mean a problem, depending upon the cause. If a murmur is heard, an ultrasound of the heart (echocardiogram) is often needed to sort it out. When I hear a murmur I will mention it and ask if it is "known." If the murmur has already been investigated, and proper action taken, then very well. If not, I will schedule testing, or see that it is arranged. The heart rate and rhythm are also evaluated with the stethoscope.

When listening to the lungs the quality of air movement is considered Good and symmetrical air flow is normal. Depth and rate are observed.

The three abnormal breath sounds your doctor may mention are; rales, rhonchi, and wheezes. Rales sound like fine crackles, and in fact are sometimes called crackles. Rubbing a lock of hair between thumb and forefinger right next to your ear produces the best imitation of rales. Rales indicate that there is fluid in the smallest parts of the lung, known as alveoli. Rales indicate either an increase of fluid pressure such as we will soon discuss in congestive heart failure, or pneumonia. Rhonchi are a coarser sound, and are less specific. Rhonchi often clear up after a cough, and thus often indicate secretions in the larger airways. Wheezing is a musical, squeaky sound and means that air is squeezing through narrowed airways. Wheezing is typical in asthma and chronic obstructive pulmonary disease, both of which we will discuss in this chapter.

Wheezes are difficult to hear without a stethoscope, and the sounds that cause parents to bring their child to the ER are often made by the mouth and pharynx (uppermost airway). Listening (auscultation) with the stethoscope often reveals "clear" lungs despite the audible upper airway noise in these children.

The Pulse Oximeter

In the ER, you will be tested with an instrument called a pulse oximeter. This is a relatively (widely adopted in the late 1980s) new device that measures circulating oxygen through the skin. Good blood flow to the finger, toe, or earlobe to which the probe is attached is required. If you look at the monitor, you will see a number and a "waveform." If there is adequate blood flow, the waveform should rise and fall with each heartbeat. The number, which normally is between 95 percent and 100 percent, represents the percentage of oxygen saturation. A "pulse ox" is far likelier to err on the low side than on the high side. If the waveform looks irregular or uneven, the reading is likely to be falsely low. If the number jumps around—for example, 61, 87, 91, 72, 94, 83—the right reading is at least the highest, 94 percent in this case. The pulse oximeter can miss oxygen but cannot "imagine" it.

While a useful tool, the pulse oximeter is not without limitations. In anemia, for example, blood cells may be well oxygenated, but if there are not enough blood cells, there is not enough oxygen reaching the tissue. Carbon monoxide toxicity cannot be detected by the usual pulse oximeter, though there are new models that can detect both oxygen and carbon monoxide. Carbon monoxide displaces oxygen, and thus a person who is suffering from carbon monoxide inhalation can be hypoxic and still have a normal pulse oximeter reading.

We will divide the causes of shortness of breath into (1) pulmonary, (2) cardiac, and (3) other.

This is a very important chapter because the majority of people I see who are truly in immediate danger of dying are either short of breath or soon will be.

Chapter 38 Shortness of Breath

Pulmonary Causes of Shortness of Breath

One of my surgical professors during residency, Dr. Felix Batistella, told me when I was an intern that the most important vital sign was the respiratory rate. Standing by the patient's bedside, Dr. Batistella would watch the patient with us. If he or she was breathing at a normal rate, and to a normal depth, it was very reassuring. If he or she was not breathing normally, there was always something seriously wrong. Since the rotation was trauma surgery, usually it was something we could fix and needed to fix right away!

If you are watching your child or a friend asleep, note the normal breathing rate. It is easiest to watch the chest rise and fall, counting on the rise. If your spouse is snoring, measuring the respiratory rate will be easy! For adults it is usually in the range of ten to fifteen breaths per minute. Often the number stated as average is twelve breaths per minute. Compared to the heart rate, it is hard to accurately measure something so slow. I say this because the heart rate and respiratory rate are usually measured over fifteen seconds and then multiplied by four to get the rate per minute. If the respiratory rate is twelve per minute, only three breaths are expected during the fifteen-second period. Missing one or adding one, depending on the period counted, makes a bigger percentage difference than missing one of the fifteen to twenty heartbeats that fall during the same period. During triage in the ER, the patient will be somewhat tense and also will have just walked a bit to get from the car to the room, so the rates average higher. Generally, we consider twenty per minute and under to be normal and over twenty breaths per minute to be abnormal for an adult.

Children breathe faster. A normal respiratory rate for a newborn is thirty to forty breaths per minute (about twice the adult rate, or a bit more). At three to six years of age, the rate has slowed to twenty to thirty per minute, and by the teens, the adult rate is reached.

Medical Wisdom

A fever will cause an increase in both heart rate and respiratory rate. I was taught that for each half-degree Celsius increase in temperature, the heart rate will increase by 10 beats per minute. For example, normal temperature is 37 degrees Celsius (which equals 98.6 Fahrenheit). If the normal heart rate is 80 per minute and the temperature is raised to 40 degrees Celsius (three degrees increase equals six half-degree increases) the heart rate will increase to 140 per minute (6 times 10 equals 60 plus 80). In my clinical experience, this is surprisingly accurate. The change in respiratory rate with fever is similar in magnitude, with a one-degree Celsius increase producing an increase in respiratory rate of five to seven breaths per minute. The change is greater in infants and small children, of course. Fever basically turns up the metabolism.

Knowing the above facts will help you decide if there is something wrong with your child's or friend's breathing.

For example, you count your ill fifteen-year-old boy's respiratory rate and find it is 28 and his (fever) temperature is 39 degrees. Since he is uncomfortable, you choose to give him 600 milligrams of ibuprofen. Measuring his temperature an hour later shows it to have decreased to 37.5. At that point his respiratory rate has decreased to 18, and he is sleeping more soundly. Since the respiratory rate is now normal, and decreased as expected with the decrease in temperature, his lungs are working fine. If his temperature decreased from 39 to 37.5 but his respiratory rate was still 25 per minute, pneumonia or another lung infection should be suspected, and a trip to the ED or doctor's office for an X-ray would be a good idea.

Shortness of breath is certainly always caused by exertion. Anyone who runs will need to breathe faster to make up for the increased oxygen demand. The important question, though, is, "Are you more short of breath than usual?" If an elderly person with COPD (chronic obstructive pulmonary disease—see also the "Cough" chapter) can usually walk to the mailbox without being short of breath but now is short of breath with that walk, discovering what has changed is the doctor's job.

Causes of shortness of breath directly related to the lungs include asthma, COPD, pneumonia, other pulmonary infections, airway obstruction, pneumothorax, pulmonary fibrosis, and pulmonary effusion.

Asthma is the exaggerated tendency of the airways to protect the lungs by constricting. We discussed asthma in the "Cough" chapter since cough is a common symptom of asthma. Everyone has the ability to have an "asthmatic reaction," which consists of wheezing, difficulty moving air in and out (especially out), and coughing. Some people have the tendency to have more "reactive" airways than others. There are chemicals that will cause anyone to have an "asthma" attack. Things that cause an asthmatic reaction are known as "triggers." A viral illness is a common trigger for an asthmatic exacerbation (attack). Sometimes certain pollens will cause a flare, as can pet dander, exercise, or cold air exposure.

Wheezing is the trademark sound of asthma. Wheezing, which is a musical squeaking produced in the airways, can be heard easily with a stethoscope, but without a stethoscope, it is sometimes hard to distinguish wheezing from other sounds. Upper airway (mouth and throat) noises, as well as nasal sounds, can be and often are mistaken for the wheezing of asthma.

Asthma is treated initially with an inhaler or nebulizer treatment (looks like smoking a water-vapor pipe) that is designed to dilate the airways. Albuterol is a typical bronchodilator, and an Albuterol inhaler is known as a "rescue inhaler." These bronchodilators work in the same way that epinephrine (adrenaline) works, opening up the breathing passages to allow more airflow. Albuterol also stimulates the heart in the same way adrenaline does, causing an increase in heart rate and in force of heart contraction, which is felt as a pounding heart by most people.

There is a relatively new rescue inhaler that has less heart activity and may be better for people with heart problems. This new inhaler, known as Xopenex, is more expensive. The only downside of the new bronchodilator is that because the telltale heart pounding is absent, it is harder to tell if a normal dose of medicine is being delivered.

Inhalers are often supplied with aero chambers known as "spacers." A spacer is a chamber into which the inhaler discharges. Spacers are especially good for children and for adults who have difficulty with the timing of inhaler use. Albuterol has a bitter taste, and children will naturally try to avoid breathing it until they realize it helps them.

The other class of inhaler contains corticosteroids, which are strong anti-inflammatory agents. Steroid inhalers act to decrease the sensitivity of the airways and to decrease the amount of secretions. Steroid inhalers are not rescue inhalers. They work over the course of days, rather than in minutes. I have had many patients come in after mistaking their steroid inhaler for their Albuterol (rescue) inhaler and suddenly realizing that "the inhaler is not working!" The idea of the steroid inhaler is to administer a small amount of steroid (anti-inflammatory) directly to the airways. After a few days of steroid inhaler use, the rescue inhaler should be needed less frequently.

Since the inhaler bottle is made of metal, it is hard to tell when it is empty. A puff of air will still come out, even after the liquid medicine is gone. To test your inhaler, detach the bottle from the plastic fitting and drop it in a cup of water. When full it should sink or float in an up-and-down position nearly below the surface of the water. When half full it will float higher and on its side, and when empty it will float on the side, and very high.

Chapter 38 Shortness of Breath

Using an Inhaler

When using an inhaler, first breathe all the way out. Activate the inhaler when you start breathing in, and continue to breathe in steadily for a full breath. Hold that full breath for a few seconds at least. If you get most of the medicine by timing it correctly, you will often have a strong urge to cough while trying to hold your breath. This urge to cough is not as bad on the second puff, if taken immediately after the first. Usually the dose is "one to two puffs," and if you cough immediately while trying to hold your breath after the first dose, you will need a second puff.

If inhaler therapy alone is not enough, oral steroids can be used to bring severe asthma under control. A five- or six-day course of prednisone is often used. The dose will likely be forty or sixty milligrams per day, taken in the morning. A short-term course of prednisone can work miracles and does not cause the adverse effects associated with long-term oral steroids. Generally, a steroid inhaler will be started as the short course of prednisone comes to an end.

We discussed COPD (chronic obstructive pulmonary disease) in detail and pneumonia briefly in the "Cough" chapter.

COPD causes chronic shortness of breath. COPD is similar to asthma, but there is permanent, irreversible lung destruction in COPD, whereas with asthma the lungs are normal in function and anatomy between acute attacks. COPD also results in wheezing, but the rescue inhalers rarely are "miracle drugs" the way they are with asthma. More steroids are generally needed, and sometimes they are needed on a regular basis. If an older, long-term smoker develops "asthma," it is usually actually COPD and is thus harder to vanquish. People with COPD are more prone to pneumonia and bacterial bronchitis, as well as cancer and lung rupture. The destruction of lung membranes from smoking we discussed in the "Cough" chapter can lead to air leaking from one of the new large air pockets into the space between the lung and chest wall, resulting in lung collapse, which is known as pneumothorax. Pneumothorax is a serious problem that we will discuss later in this chapter and again in the "Trauma" chapter. Managing COPD is a challenge, and if smoking continues, the problems only continue to worsen.

When Lung turns to "Liver"

Pneumonia differs from the lung inflammation present with a cold. Pneumonia, as it is usually discussed, is considered to be a bacterial infection. Pneumonia is a serious problem that leads to many deaths. A number of different types of bacteria cause pneumonia, and identification of the specific cause is important for treatment. Viral infections can also cause lung inflammation, which is generally referred to as pneumonitis.

Pneumonia is an acute inflammation of the lung or lungs that is so severe, the lung goes from the consistency of a fluffy sponge to a heavy, solid consistency similar to that of liver. As a matter of fact, the lung change seen on pathology (cut-up lung after death) is called "hepatization" (hepatic: liver). The spongy, inflatable lung is good for exchanging oxygen, but the blood- and infection-filled, liver-like lung of pneumonia is not. Even with thorough antibiotic treatment, pneumonia that shows up on a chest X-ray will still be visible on an X-ray a month later, and some shortness of breath will still be present a month later as well.

Pneumonia is overdiagnosed at times. Often any visible change on the chest X-ray is called "pneumonia." If your doctor diagnoses you or your child with pneumonia, it is worth asking, "How serious is the pneumonia?" A real pneumonia, which is easily visible on the chest X-ray, causes pain, shortness of breath, and is usually estimated to have a 5–15 percent mortality rate. A "common cold type" virus can cause some minor change on an X-ray, but these will resolve quickly and generally without lung damage. Changes in breathing pattern and failure to take a deep breath can also cause some minor changes in the X-ray that can be "over read" as pneumonia. In both of these cases, antibiotics may be prescribed as a precaution, and the diagnosis of pneumonia may be a fair excuse, but in actuality no pneumonia exists. The X-ray will be clear on repeat within a week or two—not the case with pneumonia.

Pneumonia typically causes cough, fever—often with intermittent shaking chills—pain with breathing, and shortness of breath. Air hunger may come at rest when pneumonia is severe or with activity if less severe.

Pneumonia can follow a viral illness. In that scenario, the typical productive cough that follows a cold will become painful, fevers will return, and the sputum will often change color or become bloody.

Whether or not a person seen in the ED and diagnosed with pneumonia needs to be admitted to the hospital depends on a variety of factors. These factors can be divided into those related to the patient and those related to the pneumonia. A number of pneumonia-severity scoring systems have been developed to determine the need for admission to the hospital and likelihood of death or serious complications from pneumonia. The CURB-65 score is one of the simpler ones. C stands for confusion; a confused patient earns a point. U stands for urea (a measure of kidney function and hydration), and a higher-than-usual level earns a point. R stands for respiratory rate; if the respiratory rate is over thirty per minute, a point is added. B stands for blood pressure; a measurement with the systolic less than ninety or diastolic less than sixty earns a point. Age greater than sixty-five earns a point. As you can see, five points are possible. Confusion and low blood pressure are signs of systemic infection and immune system overwhelm.

A well-hydrated thirty-year-old with normal vital signs and a normal respiratory rate earns no points. The CURB-65 score predicts less than a 1 percent chance of mortality at thirty days. He should be treated with oral antibiotics and sent home from the ER.

A confused seventy-year-old with a respiratory rate of thirty-five per minute and a normal blood pressure and normal labs earns three points. The CURB-65 score at three points predicts a 17 percent chance of death within thirty days. That patient requires hospitalization and probably needs the Intensive Care Unit (ICU). A CURB-65 score of five carries a 57 percent thirty-day mortality rate.

As you can see, pneumonia, despite antibiotics, remains a serious diagnosis. The transformation of fluffy, air-filled lung to "liver density lung" also causes damage and scarring of the lung in the same way that smoking causes lung damage. The difference: the damage caused by smoking is spread over many years, whereas the collateral damage to the lung as the battle against infection is fought occurs over a shorter period of time and to a more limited section of lung.

Aspiration and Choking

Aspiration of stomach contents can cause pneumonia in the very young, the very old, and those who experience a period of decreased level of alertness, such as when getting very drunk, passing out, and vomiting. Aspiration pneumonia can also occur with general anesthesia in the medical setting, and great precautions are taken to decrease the chance of aspiration. There are time limits between eating and surgery and shorter limits between liquid intake and surgery to ensure the stomach is empty. Special antibiotics such as Clindamycin are needed if aspiration is suspected to cover the "tough" bacteria we discussed in the "Bites and Stings" chapter.

Aspirating an object occurs most commonly in children, but also sometimes at the dinner table. Everyone is familiar with the need to keep small objects away from infants and toddlers. If a child is playing with small toys and suddenly begins to cough and wheeze, aspiration should be suspected. Your pediatrician and emergency physician will always suspect aspiration when treating young children with sudden onset of shortness of breath. An aspirated object, if it blocks the entire airway, will cause immediate severe distress.

You have probably seen the Heimlich maneuver on TV numerous times. The rule is to let the person try to cough and continue to try to cough up the obstruction, as long as they are able to breathe to some extent and as long as they are able to make a good effort to do so. If there is no more air movement and no effective coughing, it is time for the Heimlich maneuver. Give the person a hug from behind, placing a closed fist within the other hand at the lower chest, and give a hard, sudden squeeze. The goal is to try to "force the air out" suddenly and sharply. Repeat if needed. If this maneuver is not effective, and the person collapses to the ground, check their mouth for the object and begin CPR. An infant who aspirates is treated in a similar manner, but a single hand is enough to force the air out suddenly by applying pressure below the chest in an upward direction.

A pneumothorax is a serious cause of shortness of breath and one with which you should be familiar. Some background anatomy is needed to understand pneumothorax. The lungs are like balloons inside a box. The chest wall is the box on the sides, and the diaphragm is the bottom. The lungs are filling the entire box in the normal state. The lungs are not attached to the inside of the chest wall, but can slide freely back and forth against the smooth inside of the rib cage and diaphragm. There is a thin layer of lubricating fluid between the lungs and chest wall that is continuously recirculated. The lung is held in an inflated position by a slight negative pressure within this space.

If there is damage to the lung, so that it either bleeds or leaks air, the air or blood accumulates between the inside of the chest wall and the lung. This new fluid or air decreases lung air capacity. If there is a lot of air or fluid, the lung can collapse completely. Even worse, if the lung collapses and there is a valve effect that creates one-way flow, pressure can build, pushing on the other lung and decreasing its ability to function as well. This pressure effect is called a "tension pneumothorax." The two sides of the chest are isolated in humans, so a simple pneumothorax (collapsed lung) will not affect the other side in most cases.

The unfortunate buffalo has both sides of the chest connected, so a single hole in the chest wall will allow both lungs to collapse. Reportedly, this was why the American Indians were able to kill such a massive beast with their relatively lightweight bows. If they were able to make a hole in the buffalo's chest wall, air would enter, causing both lungs to collapse. With both lungs collapsed, the buffalo would become severely short of breath and quickly expire.

Pneumothorax can occur either spontaneously or as a result of trauma. Spontaneous pneumothorax is usually composed of air only. Traumatic pneumothorax can be either air, blood, or a combination of both, depending upon the injury. If the pneumothorax or hemothorax is large, shortness of breath can be severe, as can the resultant decrease in oxygenation. A fractured rib can puncture the lung, allowing air to escape from the lung, filling the closed space that surrounds it. A stab wound or gunshot can cause an open injury to the chest, allowing air to enter, as in the case of the buffalo, though hopefully only on one side.

For the spontaneous, air-only variety of pneumothorax, catheter removal of the air may be possible. Often a smaller pneumothorax will go away by itself without treatment, though they need to be monitored closely. If there is blood or fluid between the lung and chest wall, as in a traumatic pneumothorax or hemothorax, placement of a "chest tube," also known as a tube thoracostomy, is standard. The tube is placed laterally at about the spot where the middle of your upper arm touches the chest wall when you stand with your arm hanging at your side. The larger tube is needed to drain blood with potential clotting and to prevent recurrence of the accumulation. The tube is hooked up to a slight vacuum or a one-way valve to eliminate anything that might try to accumulate between the lung and chest wall.

A Serious Case of Pneumothorax

One of the most impressive cases of pneumothorax I have treated occurred when I was fresh out of training at the trauma center. I was working at two in the morning in the last half of a twenty-four-hour shift, and things had slowed down from the daytime rush. I was treating a fourteen-year-old female patient with an ingrown toenail. I had just performed a nerve block to anesthetize the toe for partial toenail removal when I heard a loud shouting and pounding at the glass ambulance bay doors. I looked up to see a young woman with long black hair, covered in blood from head to toe!

I jumped up and with my nurse started to help her toward the nearest bed. She was very short of breath and obviously very upset. She yelled, "It's not me, it's my husband!" She pointed toward her car in the ambulance bay. As we looked that way, her husband slid out of the car door onto the pavement. If she was covered in blood, then he was soaked.

We ran out the door and tried to help him to his feet. He was too weak, looked pale, and was very short of breath. A security guard helped us get him to the nearest bed while I continued my assessment. He was gulping mouthfuls of air, could not talk, and his eyes were wide. Listening with my stethoscope while the nurses tried to hook him up to the monitor, I heard no breath sounds on the right side and only faint breath sounds on the left. I could see that he had been stabbed in the back many times.

Grabbing a scalpel from the nearest cart, I located the place on the right chest where I would place a chest tube and quickly made the two-inch incision. Pushing my finger between the ribs, I felt the inside of the rib cage, but no lung. As I removed my finger a huge, pressurized gush of air exited the chest. The nurse standing by my right side said, "Wow!" The patient instantly took his first audible breath since he had arrived, and within seconds his color went from a pale blue to bright pink. The patient looked much better and was able to talk.

At that point I injected some local anesthetic before stitching the chest tube in place. I had used no anesthesia while making the initial incision and placing the tube, but the patient had been too close to death to notice. He now said, "Ouch," as I injected the anesthetic—it was an "ouch" I was glad to hear! I then noted his pulse oximeter to be reading 96 percent.

Listening with my stethoscope, I could hear the return of normal breath sounds on the right side, but the left was decreased. A portable chest X-ray showed the tube to be in good position on the right side and the lung fully reinflated, but there was a 30 percent pneumo/ hemothorax on the left (thirty percent of the lung cavity filled with air, rather than lung). There were multiple stab wounds to the left back as well, so this was not unexpected. I explained to the patient and his wife what had happened and that another tube would be needed on the left side. For this one I had the time to use local anesthetic first, and the tube placement went well, in the routine fashion. Pulse oximetry was then 100 percent, and supplemental oxygen was discontinued.

As the story unfolded, I learned that the man I had just treated was very well known and respected in the community. He was working at his all-night store, since an employee had called in sick, when a man walked in with a shotgun and pointed it right at his chest. The man, who was wearing a black mask, said, "Lie down on the floor." After he lay down as directed, the man set down his shotgun, pulled out a knife, straddled him, and stabbed him "many times" in the back. As the patient reported it, the stabs didn't really hurt, but felt like "slapping." The man then emptied the cash register and departed. The injured man was then able to reach a phone and call his wife.

Chapter 38 Shortness of Breath

Possibly, calling 911 would have made more sense, but his spouse was more than "up to task," and it all worked out fine in the end. All the stab wounds missed the heart and major vessels, none hit the spinal cord, and he was released from the hospital just five days later!

In this case, the cause of his severe distress was a "tension pneumothorax" of the right side, which was forcing the heart and major vessels toward the left, cutting off the use of his left lung as well. When the pressure was released, the patient experienced return of the ability to use not only the right lung, but the majority of the left, and was much relieved. Evacuating the air and blood that had leaked from the wounds in the left chest restored normal lung function.

Wear that Dust Mask!

Pulmonary fibrosis is a widespread scarring of the lung that causes shortness of breath and ongoing inflammation. A number of diseases fall under this category, and most involve the long-term inhalation of particles that cannot be broken down and absorbed by the lung. When inert substances are drawn into the lung, sometimes they cannot be expelled. In these cases the lung will either attack them or enclose them with scar tissue. Substances that are enclosed by scar tissue include sand particles, which cause "silicosis"; coal dust, which causes "anthracosis"; asbestos, which causes "asbestosis"; and so on. All of these have the same effect, which is to cause lots of small areas of lung scarring, which results in restricting the lung's ability to expand. This condition behaves similarly to COPD in many ways, and there is some overlap in both symptoms and treatment.

Intravenous drug abusers can get similar lung damage from injecting particles with their drug. "Drawing through cotton" was popular for years. The heroin was filtered with a cotton ball as it was drawn into the syringe. Small pieces of cotton were drawn into the syringe as well and when injected into any vein would flow to the right side of the heart and be pumped to the lung with the rest of the blood to be oxygenated. The pieces of cotton would not pass through the smaller vessels, but instead clog them and become areas of scarring.

Sometimes shortness of breath is increased by a pulmonary effusion. A pleural effusion occurs when the normal amount of fluid that is between the lung and chest wall/diaphragm increases, partially filling the pleural space. In the same way that a traumatic bleed or air leak causes a decrease in lung expansion, a pleural effusion, if big enough, will result in shortness of breath. The commonest cause of a pleural effusion is pneumonia. Other conditions that cause an excess amount of fluid retention, such as congestive heart failure, will cause an effusion as well. Cancer is also a frequent cause of effusion. If the cause of an effusion is not known, a sample can be withdrawn and analyzed.

Cardiac Causes of Shortness of Breath

The classic cardiac cause of shortness of breath is congestive heart failure. The heart can be weakened by many things. Age, a heart attack, long-term hypertension, a heart infection, diabetes, kidney failure, heart valve problems, and a number of other things can weaken the heart and decrease its ability to pump blood. When the heart pumps less blood (decreased cardiac output), the body's natural response is to ensure that there is plenty of blood to pump. Having enough blood ready to flow into the heart does help it to pump more out. Enough is enough, though, and the state of having too much pressure on the venous side (coming into the heart) is what causes congestive heart failure (CHF).

When there is too much pressure on the side coming into the heart, pressure builds in the lungs, and excess fluid leaks from the blood vessels and enters the breathing surfaces of the lung. This fluid interferes with the ability of oxygen to reach the blood, since the oxygen must cross the extra fluid to get to the blood. The fluid also makes it harder for the lungs to expand and move normally. Shortness of breath is the result. When people with CHF lie down, there is more pressure on the heart and lungs than when they are sitting or standing, and thus the problem worsens.

Sitting causes more pressure in the legs, and the same problem occurs there, with leg swelling called edema. The edema is most easily seen in the feet and lower legs, though as it worsens it progresses upward to involve the thighs and even the low back and abdominal wall. The fluid enters the "third body space." The fluid is outside the veins and arteries, yet not within the cells. If you press your finger firmly on the flat hard side of the shin (tibia) in a patient with edema, the finger will make a dent that remains after you remove the pressure. The dent forms as the fluid that is outside the cells and vessels moves away from the pressure. Eating salty foods, which causes water retention in most people, causes even more fluid retention in people with CHF.

New-onset CHF requires investigation to determine the cause. Blood testing will be done, as we discussed in the "Chest Pain" chapter, to see if a heart attack was the cause of the CHF. A heart attack can decrease the heart's "horse power" and thus lead to CHF. An ultrasound called an echocardiogram will be done to evaluate the heart's movement and valve function. Decreased contraction (wall movement) occurs after a heart attack, and this asymmetry of movement can be seen on the echocardiogram. A valve malfunction by itself can be enough to cause CHF. Sometimes cardiac catheterization with angioplasty, stenting, or even bypass may be needed.

Medications to optimize heart function and lifestyle changes are typically the ongoing treatment for CHF. Diuretics are still a major treatment for CHF, as you can imagine. Lasix (furosemide) is a common diuretic, and in a sensitive person with normal kidneys, it can cause liters of urine to be produced in a matter of minutes. The pressure on the heart quickly decreases, and the edema will also decrease noticeably within hours. Some of the same medications we discussed in the "Hypertension" chapter are used in the treatment of CHF. Ask your doctor about possible side effects and also about the expected result of the medications so you can know if they are effective.

It is important to know the cause of CHF. If the cause is just a generally weak heart, then medical treatment may be all that is possible. If the cause is a heart valve problem, then surgery may result in a massive improvement.

Lifestyle changes are important for the patient with CHF. Keeping track of body weight is important, both to be aware of fluid gains (rapid gains) and to lose body weight (fat) if needed to reduce the heart's workload. Avoiding salty foods and sodium-containing drinks is a good idea, since they cause water retention, which is what the patient on diuretics is fighting.

Cardiac arrhythmias can cause shortness of breath and, if they do not cause syncope (passing out) and collapse, probably cause more shortness of breath than they do chest pain. (Because of these symptoms, it was hard to decide whether to discuss arrhythmia in this chapter or in the "Chest Pain" chapter.)

Atrial fibrillation is the first arrhythmia we will discuss. Atrial fibrillation (AF) is caused by loss of the normal function of the heart's primary pacemaker: the sinus node. A chaotic, fast, and continuous series of messages to beat originates in the upper heart, and the powerful pumping part of the heart responds as often as it can to those messages.

AF is an "irregularly irregular" rhythm. In most people with AF, the rapid response of the heart is the cause of their symptoms. Either they will feel their heart racing, or they will notice that they are short of breath, either at rest or with very little exertion. When my father had his first episode of atrial fibrillation, he noticed that even climbing a flight of stairs would make him short of breath, and he could not work out at the gym as he usually did. Some people notice instantly when they go into this arrhythmia, and others cannot pinpoint when it started. Whether they notice the onset of atrial fibrillation depends in part on their heart's rate of response. Healthy hearts generally respond with a fast rate, usually in the range of 120–150 beats per minute. The rate is also highly variable and can change from 100 to 150, often in a single beat. This rapid changing of rate is what is meant by "irregularly irregular."

When a patient comes to the ER with suspected atrial fibrillation, the first step is to get an EKG to confirm. I look for obvious signs of a heart attack and for signs that the arrhythmia is causing the heart stress. Some AF patients arrive with shortness of breath and chest pain; others arrive with only the feeling of a rapid or pounding heart.

Some patients come in by ambulance, unstable, with low blood pressure, severe shortness of breath, and pain. These unstable patients need an immediate "fix," and electrocardioversion (shocking the heart back into a normal rhythm) is the answer.

If the patient is stable, with minimal symptoms, I use several medications to decrease the heart's rate of response. A calcium channel blocker (see "Hypertension" chapter) is usually my medication of first choice. Even though the rhythm is still irregular and is still AF, a slower rate allows better heart filling between contractions, and thus better function. Next is the question of whether or not to "cardiovert" the heart to a normal "sinus" rhythm.

The problem is that during a period in this irregular rhythm, a small blood clot can form in the heart, and that blood clot can break off after return to normal rhythm. The clot can then flow up through the carotid artery to the brain, causing a stroke. It takes time for a clot to form, and it is thought to be safe to cardiovert in the first forty-eight hours. Usually the onset of AF is either clear and recent, or it is unknown. If the onset is unknown or uncertain, then the rule is to anticoagulate with a blood-thinning medicine for at least several weeks before cardioversion. Coumadin (warfarin) is usually used for this blood thinning, and levels will need to be checked regularly to ensure the blood is correctly anticoagulated.

Often an additional echocardiogram (heart ultrasound) is done to look for clots. This ultrasound can be done in one of two ways. A "transesophageal" (through the mouth, with sedation/anesthesia) echocardiogram is the most accurate and reliable, but as you can imagine, less comfortable and more technically difficult. A "transthoracic" (through the chest wall) echocardiogram is easier and more comfortable, but not as trusted to find the clot. In the case of a person who cannot tolerate Coumadin, a transesophageal echocardiogram could be done and then, if no clot is present, immediate cardioversion. This could also be done if a person is tolerating AF poorly, even after rate control.

Ablation is becoming a more common procedure as a cure for recurrent arrhythmia. Ablation is done in the catheterization lab, where stenting and angioplasty are performed. The procedure involves mapping the heart's electrical pattern and then selectively burning the aberrant electrical pathway. Sometimes ablation can be very effective.

Atrial flutter is similar to atrial fibrillation (AF), but regular, rather than irregular. The rhythm center sends out regular impulses at a rate of 300 per minute. Only small children have hearts that are able to respond at 300 beats per minute, however, and most adults respond to every other impulse, with a rate of 150 per minute. Over the last ten years, the treatment of flutter has changed and is now very similar to the treatment of atrial fibrillation.

In young people, the commonest significant arrhythmia is paroxysmal supraventricular tachycardia (PSVT), which is known as a "reentry" arrhythmia. How symptomatic a person with PSVT is varies greatly. Picture an electrical loop that goes at a very fast rate. Rates are rarely as low as 120 and usually 140 or higher. Because the impulse travels in a repeating loop, it is a regular rhythm, rather than an irregular one.

Treatment is much easier than for AF, and breaking the loop even briefly will stop the arrhythmia. Sometimes changing the venous return to the heart by holding a deep breath or performing a Valsalva maneuver (breath holding with straining) will stop the arrhythmia. Activating the "vagal nerve," which we will talk about in the "Syncope and Seizure" chapter and which slows the heart, can also sometimes break the loop. Sudden immersion of the face in very cold water (45 degrees or less) can do this.

Such an immersion will slow the heart rate of a person in sinus rhythm, as well. Here in Washington state, the water in the winter is often in the low forties. My heart rate slows substantially when I first immerse my face, even though I am wearing a dive mask. Once last winter when I was entering from the beach to spear sole, I actually felt a bit dizzy. I swam back up onto the gravel beach and took my pulse. I counted eight beats in fifteen seconds. My heart rate had dropped to thirty-two beats per minute! Over about two minutes, my body adjusted, and I swam back out.

A Cause of Shortness of Breath Not to be Missed - Pulmonary Embolus

We discussed this cause of shortness of breath in the "Extremity Pain without Trauma" chapter. Blood clots called deep venous thromboses (DVT) can break off from the legs and travel to the lungs. If you have not yet read that chapter, have shortness of breath, and have not found the answer above, then reviewing that section is a good idea.

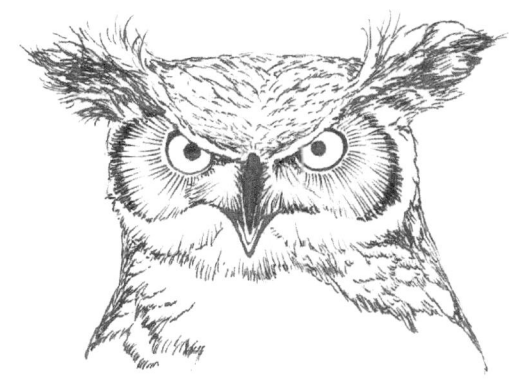

Chapter 39
Syncope and Seizure

If you're gonna collapse on a plane, I recommend business class.
The seats are bigger if you start convulsing. Although once you
pass out, it really doesn't matter.

—*Michael Westin,* Burn Notice *TV series*

Syncope is a loss of consciousness. Sometimes syncope occurs suddenly, with no warning, and sometimes there are symptoms that come first. When you come to the ER with syncope, the doctor's first goal is to decide if your syncope is caused by a dangerous problem.

Syncope caused by the heart is the primary concern. When the heart stops moving blood forward, there are only a few seconds of normal well-being, followed by a few more seconds of lightheadedness, flashing lights, and dizziness, followed by syncope. Often cardiac syncope comes so suddenly that the patient has no memory of any symptoms before awakening on the ground, often with a relatively serious injury from the fall. Feeling faint and easing oneself to the ground is very different from sudden syncope. An uncontrolled fall, with no chance to guard one's head, can cause a serious head, neck, or facial injury.

Once I treated a professional basketball player who had a true cardiac syncope while walking at mid-court. He fell (from a height of almost seven feet!), breaking his jaw and sustaining a sizable laceration.

In the "Chest Pain" chapter, you learned that a common manifestation of acute myocardial infarction (heart attack) is sudden death. The sudden death is a cardiac syncope without spontaneous recovery. Nothing to mess with, eh? The cause of sudden death, to be sudden, needs to be an instant and complete change, and in this case the change is to the heart's rhythm.

The most feared arrhythmia is ventricular fibrillation. When ventricular fibrillation (VF) occurs, the heart immediately stops coordinated movement and stops pumping. A heart in VF looks like a bag full of worms. There is a twitching, squirming motion of many origins, rather than the usual progressive contraction followed by relaxation. Caught early, while the heart is still well oxygenated, ventricular fibrillation can be converted back to sinus in most cases. This is why AEDs (automated external defibrillators) are so successful, compared with medics who arrive five or ten minutes later. This is also why the precordial thump (which we discussed earlier) is often successful—it is immediate. Though a precordial thump only generates ten to fifteen joules of electricity, while an AED generates several hundred joules, a small shock is often enough during those first few critical seconds. More electricity is needed as time passes, and eventually no amount will convert the dying heart to a functional rhythm.

Chapter 39 Syncope and Seizure

The other arrhythmia that causes sudden cardiac death is ventricular tachycardia (VT). Unlike VF, VT is an organized rhythm, but originating in the ventricle (the thick, muscular, pumping lower part of the heart) and very fast. Some people can tolerate it, and in those cases it may even be "stable," with few symptoms. Other people cannot tolerate VT, and forward flow is inadequate. Some people can tolerate VT in a recumbent position, but cannot sit or stand up without dizziness and syncope. The brain is higher than the heart while standing/sitting, but closer to the same level when lying down, and thus less blood pressure is needed to reach the brain and maintain consciousness.

A Witnessed Cardiac Syncope

The first cardiac syncope I personally witnessed was during my second year as an emergency medicine resident. I was treating a seventy-one-year-old woman who had fallen in the kitchen. Her husband had been in the living room and heard her head hit the ground with a loud "thump." She did not respond to his voice, so he went into the kitchen and found her on the floor in a "pool of blood." He called 911. The paramedics found her fully recovered, standing in the kitchen and holding pressure on her left eyebrow, where there was a two-centimeter laceration and swelling.

I did a neurologic exam and found no problems. Her EKG was normal, but I kept her on the monitor. She had lived for seventy-one years and had never passed out before. She remembered nothing before waking up on the floor with "sticky red stuff on my face." She said this with a smile and laugh as she rubbed her red fingers together to show me. I had sent labs and was planning to admit her to the hospital for continued monitoring. I anesthetized her laceration with lidocaine, and my tech irrigated the wound. I saw that she was in a normal rhythm on the monitor as I put on my sterile gloves. I told her I was going to place a "drape" over her face so that only her wound would show.

Just as I reached for her with the drape, her eyes rolled back, her mouth opened with a moan, and she slumped. Her monitor sounded an alarm! I looked at the monitor; she had changed to the closely spaced "saw-tooth" waves of ventricular tachycardia! The thought that went through my mind, and I still remember it clearly was, "No you don't!" I dropped the drape and gave her a hard precordial thump; instantly she went back into sinus rhythm. Within three seconds she said, "What happened?"

I called her nurse and asked her to print out a strip from the monitor recording. The strip showed a sudden transition from normal sinus rhythm to ventricular tachycardia. I asked the patient's nurse to give a hundred milligrams of lidocaine IV. Lidocaine is an antiarrhythmic. When injected into a wound, lidocaine causes anesthesia by stopping nerve conduction, and when given intravenously, the lower concentration has a similar effect, slowing conduction. In this case the slower conduction would hopefully stop the "runaway" conduction that caused the arrhythmia.

I waved for my attending. He had narrowly missed the action, but was now at the nursing station. My attending, myself and a medical student were examining the strip when the nurse arrived with the lidocaine. We explained to the patient what had happened, showed her the strip, and let her know that we now knew why she had fallen at home. I also let her know that she was definitely staying in the hospital.

I got a new drape, put on new sterile gloves, and was just opening the drape when…eeeee, the alarm! Once again her eyes rolled back, and she went limp. Once again I dropped the drape and gave a fast precordial thump, and thankfully once again she went right back to sinus rhythm and woke up. "What happened, did you hit me?" were her first words this time. I was more prepared the second time and probably gave the thump a second or two sooner, so she had some memory of it. By this time, the nurse was just giving the lidocaine. We added a lidocaine drip, and her heart behaved until she left the ED for a monitored bed on the hospital floor about two hours later. While she waited, she discussed with the cardiology fellow surgery to place an internal defibrillator/pacemaker.

With a cardiac syncope you will first have an EKG to see if the cause is an arrhythmia. Sometimes there are hints on the EKG that indicate a heart rhythm problem could be coming and going. Since the EKG is—when it comes to detecting arrhythmias—only a "snapshot" of the heart, you will be placed on a cardiac monitor. If your story or the EKG/monitor is suspicious for an arrhythmia, you will need to either be admitted to the hospital for further monitoring, or if the suspected arrhythmia is a nonlethal one, a Holter monitor can be used to record your heart activity for a longer time. A Holter monitor is a small mobile monitor you can wear under your clothes for an extended period. Holter monitoring equipment is getting smaller and more and more effective. Your doctor or cardiologist will then analyze the information from the monitor.

Vasovagal Syncope – "Fainting"

A common cause of syncope among healthy people is seeing their own blood or the blood of others. This sort of syncope is called "vasovagal syncope." The vagal nerve is part of the autonomic nervous system. In general, the job of the autonomic nervous system is to regulate pulse rate and blood pressure, as well as other physiologic functions. Activation of the vagal nerve and the resultant decrease in heart rate, as well as withdrawal of the opposite (sympathetic) side of the autonomic nervous system, results in a decrease in heart rate and a fall in blood pressure. As we discussed earlier, less blood pressure is needed to stay conscious in the lying (recumbent) position than when standing up. If someone is seated in a chair when his or her blood is drawn and suddenly feels the warning signs of syncope (fainting), lowering the chair so the person is lying down will often prevent loss of consciousness. My editor suggested that the readers would be very interested in knowing the exact mechanism by which seeing blood causes syncope…so would your doctor! There are a number of theories, and it is clear that the upper (thinking) brain does have the potential to influence the autonomic nervous system.

Given experience, a person can learn to avoid vagal triggers. It is also possible to overcome the tendency to faint by the use of therapy or by other distraction/mind-control methods. Certainly if you feel the nausea, sweatiness, and other symptoms of a coming vasovagal syncope, lying down before you fall is a good idea.

Sometimes people will be in an upright position when they pass out. If they are standing, they will generally fall, or if they feel it coming, they will squat, kneel, or lie down. Lying down and, if possible, raising the feet and legs will help and will result in the person waking up within a minute. Full recovery is not immediate, and if the person tries to stand right away, he or she will usually feel faint again.

If you see someone about to faint, help him or her to the ground so there is no injury from falling. Then raise the person's legs and prop them up. By the time you do this, the person will normally be waking up. Next observe the person's breathing while you feel his or her pulse. The person's skin will often be moist. When you feel the pulse, the rate will often be very slow. The vagal nerve caused the person's heart rate to slow down until there was no longer enough flow to make it "uphill" to the head.

As an illustrative contrast, consider a runner I cared for who collapsed while running a marathon. It was a hot day, and I was stationed at the top of a steep hill at the end of mile 20. When I checked the runner's pulse, her heart rate was over 150. She had become dehydrated, and her heart was trying to make up for the lack of blood volume by beating faster (not slowing down, as happens in a vasovagal syncopal collapse). She felt much better after three liters of intravenous fluid.

Not a Seizure – A Syncopal Convulsion

If a person who has a vasovagal syncope is kept in an upright position, an interesting phenomenon called a "syncopal convulsion" can occur. A syncopal convulsion looks like a seizure. Generally, there will be a few seconds of jerking of both sides of the body, both arms and legs, but this is much shorter than a usual seizure. If the person does not fall down or lay down, these convulsive movements can continue. Falling or slumping so that the head is lower will restore flow to the brain and stop the convulsion.

I treated a young woman once that demonstrates the phenomena of syncopal convulsion. A police officer brought her in for a "legal blood alcohol, and medical clearance to incarcerate." He was concerned that she had faked a seizure to avoid being prosecuted for driving under the influence of alcohol (DUI). The officer once told me he saw the car driving erratically on the freeway and followed it. The car pulled over onto the shoulder and stopped. When he walked up to the window, the driver, a young woman, was apparently having a seizure. He reported that her arms and legs were "twitching around" and her eyes were "rolled back." He unbuckled her and managed to lay her over across the seat, at which time the twitching stopped. She awakened and was able to talk normally before the paramedics arrived. She was fully recovered by arrival to the ED and able to tell a good story: She was on her way home from work and was listening to a new medical thriller audio book. A part came where they were describing a needle entering a person's arm, and she always fainted when her blood was drawn! She felt herself getting sweaty and thought she might pass out, so she pulled over onto the shoulder. The next thing she remembered was the officer shaking her awake, and then trying to sit up. She had passed out and was held in an upright position by her seat belt. Being upright prevented the blood from getting to her brain, and the result was the syncopal convulsion that the officer witnessed.

The fact that she was able to recall almost the entire incident means it was not a seizure. The officer remained at bedside, despite my explanation, until the alcohol level returned at zero.

Seizure –Electrical Storm in the Brain

Seizures look very impressive and very dangerous, but in general they look a lot more dangerous than they are. Most people with recurrent seizures consider them to be a part of life. They recover uneventfully, deal with any injuries, and continue living.

Seizures can be generalized, which means they involve both sides of the brain and therefore both sides of the body, or they can be partial. A partial seizure can be limited to a small section of the brain, and if it involves the movement (motor) part of the brain, will only cause movement on one side. A partial seizure is usually remembered by the patient, whereas a generalized seizure is not.

Seizures are essentially a self-perpetuating "electrical storm" of the brain. The aberrant electrical activity starts in a single location and then propagates. If it propagates across the lower areas of the brain to reach the other motor cortex (so that both sides of the body are involved), the storm has to pass through the centers of more basic brain function, wiping out any recent memories, stopping the creation of new memories, and rendering the person unconscious.

Names have been given to some kinds of seizures. "Grand mal" is often used to describe a generalized "tonic clonic" (tightness and movement) seizure. Grand mal literally means "big bad," since that is how a grand mal seizure looks. "Absence" (pronounced absanze) seizures are brief moments of disconnection from consciousness, sometimes with staring or chewing. This condition is mostly diagnosed in patients ages four to twelve years, and often resolves spontaneously. There are other types of seizure/attack as well. These are general groupings, and each seizure is unique, and each patient with seizures needs to be considered individually.

Chapter 39 Syncope and Seizure

As stated above, patients with a generalized seizure have a loss of consciousness and do not remember anything from the period before the seizure (usually about fifteen minutes) or the period after (also usually about fifteen minutes). The period during which the patient is confused and disoriented after the seizure is known as the post-ictal period. The duration of the post-ictal period varies from patient to patient, and to some extent increases with the duration of the seizure.

At the university we treated a fair number of homeless patients with recurrent seizure, and I noted some interesting phenomena. Patients with tonic clonic seizures (grand mal) would often report remembering everything that happened during a seizure. As I explained above, that is not possible. After several years, a patient took me into his confidence and explained that "if they think you won't remember, they'll roll ya and rob ya blind."

Sometimes a patient has an "aura" before their seizure. One patient, a twenty-nine-year-old woman, told me she "smelled burning rubber" just before a seizure. Her seizures most likely originated in the part of the brain responsible for smell. I explained to her on our first visit that people with her kind of seizure (grand mal) generally don't remember anything for fifteen minutes before and fifteen minutes after the seizure. She insisted that she "smelled burning rubber" just before the seizure. I was intrigued and asked a series of questions. After a bit of digging, it turned out that she couldn't actually remember the smell, but whenever she had a seizure, her friends would tell her that right before the seizure, she would say something like, "Do you smell burning rubber? I smell something bur…," and the seizure would begin. Her friends always told her about the "burning rubber" after her recovery, and she then knew her aura without actually ever being able to remember it! When she started talking about burning rubber, her friends knew to move her gently away from dangerous objects and to have her lie down.

Medical Wisdom

Probably the commonest seizure patient we see in the ER is a person with a long history of seizures. Even with antiseizure (anti-epileptic) medication, seizures often still continue to occur, though hopefully at a much lower frequency. The patient is walking along, and the next thing he remembers, he is in an ambulance arriving at the ER. If he had the seizure at home, or when he was with friends who understood his epilepsy, he most likely would not have come in. It is hard to blame a bystander for calling 911. When someone suddenly falls to the pavement, shaking all over, drooling, and having difficulty breathing, what else can you do? It is worth looking for a medic alert bracelet, though none may be present.

Some epileptic patients have a known cause of their seizures, and in other cases it is idiopathic (no discoverable cause). Seizures can follow head injuries and other forms of brain damage. They can also be associated with drug and alcohol withdrawal and abuse.

If you see a person fall to the ground and have involuntary movements or tightness, go over to him or her and ensure that he or she will not be harmed by hitting nearby objects. Prevent the person from accidentally falling into the road, into water, or off a cliff, depending on the situation. If the person is not moving too violently, roll him or her onto the left side, as it is harder to aspirate vomit when in that position.

Seizures usually only last a minute or two, though they seem much longer. Seizures I witness are treated with a benzodiazepine (generally Ativan), usually stop quickly, and rarely recur. There are many antiseizure medications with varying side effects and efficacy.

If a seizure continues for more than twenty or so minutes, it is considered "status epilepticus." Exhaustion of the brain cells can result in damage, and increasingly powerful measures are taken to stop the seizure as time passes. Eventually the brain can be "put to sleep" with barbiturates to give it rest.

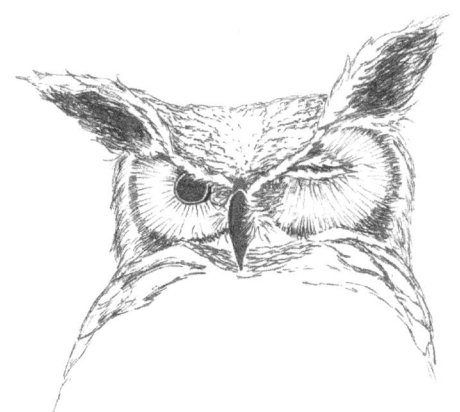

Chapter 40
Trauma

Reject your sense of injury and the injury itself disappears.

—Marcus Aurelius

The subject of trauma is broad, and this book has already covered much of it. In the "Bites and Stings" chapter, we covered punctures and infection. We have talked about blood loss and many blood tests useful in trauma. In the "Head Injury" chapter, we discussed head injury in detail. In the "Death and Dying" chapter we reviewed some deaths by trauma. Coming up in the "Wounds and Wound Repair" chapter, we will discuss wound repair and treatment as well as review some principles of infection and infection prevention. This chapter would be very long if it had to cover the entire subject of trauma.

When one thinks of the emergency department, it is natural to think of trauma. We do see a lot of both minor and major trauma. Some emergency departments are designated as a "trauma center." These centers are further divided into levels depending on their capability. The teaching hospital University of California Davis in Sacramento, which I have often referred to in this book, is a "level one trauma center." A small hospital with incomplete specialty services might be a level three or four trauma center. Regulations specify which level a facility is granted.

Paramedics will preferentially take a trauma victim to a trauma center. For a hospital in a big city, being designated a level one or two trauma center is a mixed blessing. Many of the people who are shot, stabbed, and otherwise assaulted have no insurance. Some of them are earning their income through, shall I say, methods that are not easily tracked by the IRS. Much of their business tends to be in cash. Treating the patients from violent trauma can transform a peaceful emergency department into a dangerous place. On the other hand, many people with insurance/means of payment are involved in falls and motor vehicle accidents (MVAs).

Blunt Trauma vs. Penetrating

Trauma is often classified as either blunt or penetrating. Trauma centers in affluent areas tend to see blunt trauma, mostly caused by MVAs and falls. Trauma centers in urban areas see more of the penetrating variety, sometimes referred to as the "knife and gun club." In the "Shortness of Breath" chapter, we went over a case of stabbing. In the "Death and Dying" chapter, we discussed several cases of blunt abdominal trauma, with liver injury and death.

In general, blunt trauma is considered more "challenging and interesting" by emergency physicians. When I applied for my residency training in emergency medicine I asked about the percentage of blunt versus penetrating trauma. I wanted to be sure I wouldn't be seeing an endless stream of gunshots and stab wounds. I was assured that in Sacramento there would be a good mix of blunt and penetrating injuries. On my first night as an intern, I personally treated eleven gunshot victims! Luckily, that night was an exception.

As a shooter and hunter I had a special interest in the gunshot victims. Some things I noted as I treated hundreds of gunshot victims were interesting. I saw many bullets on X-ray. The bullets were all shaped like the classic "bullet shape," without deformation. I saw one frangible (fragmenting) round in the shoulder of a prisoner that had escaped from Folsom Prison and been apprehended, but otherwise it was very rare to see an expanded "hollow point" type bullet on X-ray. I also never treated a "center mass" hit with a rifle. Those victims die on the scene. Gang members seem to buy cheap ammunition. I think they are after "the most bang for the buck." The commonest gunshot injury by far was partial penetration with a 9 mm. solid lead bullet. Most of these patients had treatable injuries and survived. I treated many shotgun victims, but there were no patients that survived a center mass hit with buckshot if fired from within about 20 yards or a birdshot hit within about 20 feet.

Hunters can appreciate the incredible degree of tissue damage done by a high speed bullet. The extensive damage seen when field dressing a rifle shot deer is essentially never seen in the ER.

If a bullet is seen during evaluation, it is removed. Otherwise it is not standard practice to "dig around" to try to find bullets. If there is suspicion that the bullet is impinging upon vital structures, or is near major vessels, into which it may erode, it may be removed.

Major and Minor Trauma

Trauma is also divided into major and minor trauma. The division here is less clear-cut than the blunt/penetrating division. For example, when we get a radio call about a fall, we need to decide whether it is a dangerous fall that should be classified as major trauma or a minor fall. At UCD, a fall was considered major trauma if it was from a height of greater than nineteen feet. At that height, a fall is not only likely to break leg and arm bones, but could break the spine, damage internal organs, or injure the chest wall. The monkey bars at school, for example, cause numerous forearm fractures, but I have not yet seen a spleen or liver rupture (not that it is impossible) from a fall off the bars. Falling down a flight of twenty one-foot-tall stairs does not equal a single twenty-foot fall. The decision to classify a patient as a victim of major trauma also has to do with the patient's condition. For example, a fall from twelve feet with neck pain and paralysis resulting would be classified as major trauma. If a patient is classified as major trauma, a more complete trauma team is assembled before the patient arrives.

Great efforts are taken by firefighters and medics to immobilize the spine after trauma. Almost everyone taken to the trauma center is immobilized on a rigid "backboard," with the neck given additional protection. This is an extremely uncomfortable and potentially damaging situation for patients, and hopefully they are assessed and some or all of the restraints are removed shortly after arrival at the ED. These efforts at immobilization are taken to prevent further injury during transport. In medical school we were immobilized on backboards as a learning experience, and within a few minutes, I was uncomfortable; after fifteen minutes I was in pain, which became worse for the next half hour. During the second thirty minutes, I went back and forth between numbness and pain as I tried, without success, to shift position to re-establish blood flow. By the end of the hour, I swore I would never force one of my patients to undergo what I had just been through. Unfortunately, sometimes immobilization is required, but in the vast majority of cases, absolute immobilization can be relaxed on arrival at the ED.

Chapter 40 Trauma

Motor vehicle accidents (MVAs), now more often referred to as motor vehicle collisions (MVCs), are classified according to the speed and point of impact. For example, a low-speed rear-end MVA might be less than ten miles per hour, with bumper damage only. A "high-speed front-impact MVA with passenger intrusion" indicates severe damage, with the passenger space being entered by a part of the car that does not belong there. "Intrusion" converts an MVA into a direct-impact experience and greatly increases the chance of serious injury. A "high-speed passenger-side T-Bone MVA" may cause intrusion into the passenger space and potential death from direct impact. If the patient was the driver in the same accident, he or she would be expected to be less severely injured than the passenger.

Children's car seats should be placed in the center of the back seat, which decreases the chance of an impact causing "intrusion into the child's space."

When treating a victim of trauma, the same initial steps—"airway, breathing, circulation," or ABC—are taken as with other seriously ill patients. When you approach a person who has suffered trauma, ask him or her a question, such as, "Are you OK?" If the person can respond and appears to be breathing normally, you have done A and B. If the person does not respond, note the condition of the face, oropharynx (mouth, teeth, tongue, throat), and neck.

If the neck is in a bad position, it may need to be straightened. Do this by moving around to the top of the person's head and placing a hand on each side, over the ears. While supporting the weight of the head, gently move the head to a neutral position, with the neck straight. If the neck is broken, you may or may not see swelling and other changes. Know that injury has already occurred and that the gentle movement you perform is needed. Further injuries occur very rarely. Another key to avoiding further injury is to apply traction—pulling gently to make the neck longer rather than shorter—as you return it to a neutral position. The primary purpose of a cervical collar is to hold the neck to length and not allow shortening.

If there is a broken jaw or other oral injury, you may need to help the breathing by moving the jaw. A "jaw thrust" in which, while you are still behind the patient's head, you gently move the jaw forward (upward) can help to open the airway.

"C" for circulation comes next, so feel for the person's pulse. If the person is talking and awake, they have at least some blood pressure. If they are lying down, however, it may be only 60/40.

Estimating blood pressure "in the Field"

The next three paragraphs are a review from the "Anemia" chapter.

The first location to feel a pulse is the radial artery. To find the radial artery, feel on the soft (under) side of the wrist, on the thumb (radial) side about an inch toward the elbow from the wrist crease. Press hard enough to partially block the blood flow, and you should feel it easily. The radial pulse is a common place to check, but as the blood pressure drops, it will be one of the first to decrease in strength.

The carotid pulse is strong, easy to find, and can be felt even if the blood pressure is low. To find the carotid pulse, take the index and long fingers of your right hand and lay them flat across the left side of your neck at the level of the "Adam's apple," known medically as the thyroid cartilage. Your thumb will be on the right side of the windpipe (trachea). Press in with the flattened fingers and you will feel the pulse. The pulse is easier to feel higher on the neck, than lower. The carotid pulse is a good one to check while you are on a treadmill, and is the one you will feel for if you examine an unconscious person.

The femoral pulse is harder to find on oneself than the others, because of the angle. To find the femoral pulse on another person, lay the flats of your fingers along the hip crease, and press hard enough to partially occlude the femoral artery.

There are some rules you can use to quickly estimate blood pressure. Find the carotid (neck) pulse. If a carotid pulse is felt, the systolic (top number) blood pressure is as a rule at least 60. If you can feel a femoral pulse, the systolic pressure is at least 70, and if you can feel a radial artery (wrist) pulse, the systolic blood pressure is at least 80. While you are checking the pulse, observe the patient's body for signs of bleeding and make note of any obvious injuries. If there is visible bleeding, control it either by direct pressure or by tourniquet.

The next step is to examine the chest and abdomen. You may have already noticed, or the patient may have mentioned, some injuries to those areas by now. If not, the patient may be in luck. Injuries to the chest and abdomen are the trickiest and potentially deadly.

Observe the chest. Is the left side moving the same as the right? Is the person breathing normally or faster than normal? Are there red marks, swellings, or other visible signs of injury?

Pushing on (palpation of) the chest is the next step. Start by pushing on the clavicles and rechecking the lower neck. Clavicle fractures are common, and unless accompanied by rib fractures or other injury are usually not a serious problem. Most clavicle fractures, even displaced ones, are most often treated with only a sling and pain medicine. Clavicle fractures can be very painful, though, and will need pain treatment. Sometimes a clavicle fracture can be associated with another, more serious injury.

Palpate the ribs and sternum both on the sides and front of the chest. Note any rib pain, bruising, swelling, and any strange "crunchy" feelings. An unstable fractured rib can have a strange "popping" feel to it. If a rib has punctured the lung, there is often air beneath the skin, which is referred to as crepitus. There is nothing else that feels quite like air where it doesn't belong, and it is hard to describe beyond saying that it feels "crunchy." If there is crepitus, it is almost certain that a chest tube (see "Shortness of Breath" chapter) will be needed on that side of the chest.

If a person with chest trauma and crepitus is short of breath, or becomes short of breath, and no chest tube is available, there are several other options. You know that removing the blood and/or air from the space between the lung and chest wall is what needs to be done. Just making the chest-tube incision may be enough to relieve the pressure. Remember the case of "tension pneumothorax" from stabbing? It was my incision between the ribs that allowed the pressurized air to escape from the chest, reexpanding the lung. By the time the chest tube was inserted, the man was already breathing much better. If it is air that is causing the pressure, an IV catheter can allow the air to escape. The catheter can then be used to allow air to escape at intervals. Blood will not be removed well with such a catheter, though. George Clooney in the movie *We Three Kings* uses such a catheter arrangement to drain a pneumothorax. An internal camera view shows the collapsing lung when SFC Barlow is shot in the chest, and his lung begins to collapse as air enters the space between the lung and chest wall. Though not a movie for kids, it is a basically accurate depiction of an important emergency technique.

Rib Fractures

Rib fractures are a common injury, and even if not associated with more serious internal injury, are very painful and can cause problems. If, while you are palpating the chest, you find a tender area, and if pushing on the rib at that location causes a sharp pain, you have likely found a rib fracture. Rib fractures are a bit tricky, since they do not always show up well on X-rays. Each rib is surrounded by tough fibrous tissue, and the muscles between the ribs also give them support. A rib can be badly broken, yet spring back into perfect position and stay there. It is this spontaneous return to normal position that makes a "nondisplaced" rib fracture very hard to see on an X-ray. A "displaced" rib fracture is much easier to see on a chest X-ray. They are also easy to see on X-ray years later, long after they are completely healed.

If you or your loved one has a broken rib, whether seen on X-ray or diagnosed by the injury and symptoms, it is important that normal breathing be maintained. Rib-fracture pain will generally last for about six weeks. Severe pain is expected for a week or so. If a person fails to take deep breaths for a period of time, areas of the lung will "stick together" a bit. This sticking together (known as atelectasis) can cause pneumonia. Enough pain medication should be prescribed to ensure that the person can take a deep breath. There is a device called an "incentive spirometer" that should be used if there is pain on breathing. The incentive spirometer measures inhalation. A plunger rises as the person inhales through a tube. Watching the plunger go up encourages deep breathing. Additional pain medication may be needed at night.

When I fell onto a boat's rail, breaking a left lower rib, I could not sleep on the left side for five weeks. For the first few days. I would awaken when I accidentally rolled onto that side. After a while I grew accustomed to not moving that way. The pain was present until the movement of bone at the site of the break stopped. The pain was literally there one day and gone the next.

The Abdomen…Tricky and Deadly after Trauma

After examining the chest, you will move to the person's abdomen. Ask if there is abdominal pain, and if the answer is yes, ask for the location. The abdomen is the trickiest part of the trauma patient, and abdominal injury is potentially deadly. If there is serious abdominal pain caused by trauma, a trip to the emergency department is mandatory. A superficial injury to the abdomen may not be serious, but injury to the abdominal organs must be excluded.

Medical Wisdom

Observe the abdomen for signs of visible injury, as you did with the chest. After a head-on (deceleration) MVA, there are often red marks from the seat belt. These may be present across the chest and by their location can show whether the person was the driver or passenger. A seat belt mark across the abdomen can indicate serious abdominal injury.

Normally, the abdomen is soft when relaxed. If there is bleeding into the abdomen, diffuse pain and severe tenderness is typical. Remember how we discussed "peritonitis" in the "Abdominal Pain" chapter? Blood irritates the peritoneum and causes pain. The abdomen will often feel "hard," as the person, either voluntarily or involuntarily, tightens the abdominal muscles. Medically we call this an "acute abdomen." If this sort of pain is present, getting the person quickly to the emergency department is essential and calling 911 an excellent idea. The medics will know to choose a trauma center, if available.

The pelvic bones are the next thing to check. The bony pelvis is a strong structure and in young people is not easily injured by a fall from standing height. In the elderly, a fall onto the hip will often break either the hip or pelvis, depending on the angle of impact. A side impact to the car door with "intrusion" can hit the pelvis directly, breaking it in a very bad way. Pushing on the bones of the pelvis, first in a downward direction, and then compressing the pelvis from both sides at the same time, should reveal tenderness if there is an injury.

You have already evaluated the neck, but returning there now is a good idea. Does the neck need to be further stabilized? Is it still in a good position? The remainder of the spine and back are harder to assess. If you have found injuries and called 911, wait until firefighters or medics arrive before moving the person.

If you must examine the back, your approach will depend partly on what you have found so far. With one person stabilizing and maintaining traction of the neck (holding it out to length), two, or better, three others roll the patient onto the less injured side, allowing someone to examine and treat the back. This technique is called a "log roll," and is how people with suspected neck and back injury are removed from the back board in the ER. The person holding the head (and applying gentle traction) will count, so everyone can work together in a synchronous fashion: "One, two, three, roll." After the hard board is removed, the shards of glass and dirt dusted from the bed, and the back examined, the count is repeated to roll the person onto the back once again.

Checking for a neurologic deficit is often cited as an important recommendation. We won't discuss this in too much detail, but asking the patient to grip and push/pull with each arm and leg is a good start. You can also ask about numbness or tingling. You will probably have already noted nerve problems, if they exist, by this time.

Spinal injury is not always obvious and not always as painful as injuries to the arms and legs. Other injuries can also distract a person from the less painful spinal injuries. For this reason, spinal injury is not often ruled out initially in the emergency department if there are other injuries. While at the university, I treated a woman who was nine months pregnant after a major motor vehicle accident. She was the driver, and the accident was a rollover. She was restrained on a backboard, with a cervical spine collar, but was not flat, since lying flat in advanced pregnancy puts pressure on the abdominal vessels.

She complained of no neck pain, but did have an abrasion to her forehead that looked like it happened on asphalt! Her ABC's were reassuring, and she had no neurologic deficit. She had an obvious bleeding, open fracture of the ankle, and that was her complaint when asked what hurt. She had no chest or abdominal pain on palpation. She complained of no neck or back pain. I anesthetized the ankle with nerve blocks and straightened it painlessly.

Medical Wisdom

Meanwhile, portable chest and lateral cervical spine X-rays were done. Back in those days, X-rays were actually pieces of plastic film, and we had a view box by the bed. The radiology tech would bring the films to us when they were developed. Now X-rays are mostly digital and the result available almost instantaneously. Since the ankle was no longer hurting, I asked her how she was doing. She said, "Now my neck is hurting…and it is bad." Her neck was still immobilized. A few minutes later, the chest and neck X-rays arrived. Her neck was broken in three places! She delivered her healthy baby two weeks later in complete cervical spine immobilization!

Alcohol can also act as an anesthetic. We often need to watch patients with a dangerously high blood-alcohol level while they "sober up." Neck X-rays are done routinely on intoxicated patients if there is any suspicion of neck injury. An example of alcohol acting as an anesthetic was presented in the "Extremity Pain after Trauma" chapter.

Certain "mechanisms of injury" are associated with particular pairings of fractures. One example is the person who jumps from a height, landing on both feet. If the weight conducts through the heel, a fracture of the heel bone(s) (calcaneous) can occur. The force is great and often conducts to the back, resulting in a fracture of the lower spine as well. There are too many of these associated injuries to go over them all; suffice it to say that following the path of force may lead to the discovery of more injuries.

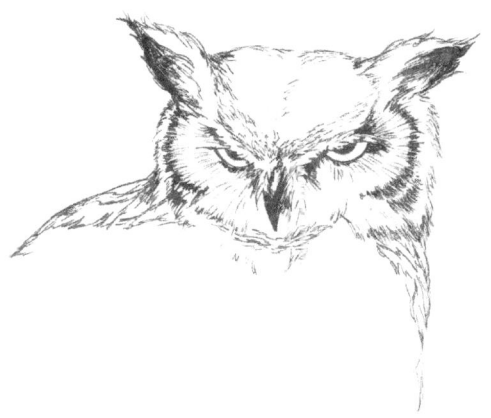

Chapter 41
Urinary Problems

I drink too much. The last time I gave a urine sample it had an olive in it.

—Rodney Dangerfield

The urinary tract is made up of the kidneys, ureters, bladder, and urethra. Common problems include infection of the bladder or kidneys, kidney stones, urinary retention, and kidney failure.

Urinary-tract infection (UTI) is certainly the commonest urinary-tract-related problem we see in the ER. The commonest urinary-tract infection is an infection of the bladder, also known as cystitis. A bladder infection is characterized by burning with urination (dysuria) and the need to urinate frequently and badly (urgency). Fever is usually not present with bladder infections, but tenderness right above the pubic bone, over the bladder, is often present.

UTIs are much commoner in females than in males. This is mostly because there is a shorter distance from the outside to the bladder, and therefore a shorter distance for bacteria to travel. There are also more bacteria around the outlet (urethral meatus) in females than in males because it is a moist area, rather than dry. Sexual activity in young women is a common cause of UTI. Women should urinate after sexual activity as this can "flush" the urethra and remove some of the bacteria. "Honeymoon cystitis" is a phrase coined to indicate the increase in urinary-tract infections in newly married women with a sudden increase in sexual activity. Contributing to honeymoon cystitis could also be the heat in a place like Hawaii, where it is easy to get dehydrated. Combining decreased urine output from dehydration with increased sexual activity is a double whammy.

The good news is that a simple UTI is easily treated with antibiotics. There is also a urinary analgesic called pyridium that helps stop most of the burning. Some think cranberry juice helps prevent infection. Certainly maintaining hydration, and thus a good flow of urine, is helpful.

If a bladder infection is allowed to persist, it can move up the ureters to the kidneys. The kidneys are located against the back of the abdominal wall near the spot where the lowest ribs join the spine. An infection of the kidneys is known as pyelonephritis, which is pronounced "pile-oh-neff-right-us." Pyelonephritis is more serious than a simple bladder infection and generally merits IV antibiotics, followed by oral antibiotics. Pyelonephritis usually causes fever, and the pain is usually felt over the affected kidney/s as well as in the bladder. A person with pyelonephritis looks and feels much sicker than a person with a simple bladder infection. Hospitalization is sometimes required.

A sexually transmitted disease should be considered, especially if burning is present and the urine is not infected. Gonorrhea causes severe burning in males, whereas chlamydia causes more itching.

Chapter 41 Urinary Problems

Both will cause some discharge (drainage, oozing) from the penis—more with gonorrhea than with chlamydia.

The frequency of UTI rises among older men because the prostate often starts causing problems with emptying the bladder. The prostate gland surrounds the urethra before it gets to the penis. The prostate gland grows with age in the same way that ears and noses grow. Since the prostate gland surrounds the tube through which the urine needs to flow, it can constrict the tube, making it harder for urine to pass. It is not uncommon for older men to have trouble emptying the bladder fully, and therefore they need to "get the top off" more frequently. The severity of nocturia (getting up to urinate at night) is rated according to how many times a man needs to get up at night to go to the bathroom. Once a night is not bad, three or more times a night is severe and disturbing to both the patient and his partner.

Often nocturia is related to sleep apnea (difficulty breathing at night, sometimes with loud snoring), rather than urinary retention. A patient with sleep apnea wakes up frequently during the night, and if he notices he has to go to the bathroom, he will get up and go. The amount voided may empty the bladder fully, unlike the case with prostatic urinary retention, but it may be done several times in a night. If you have, or think your partner has, a problem with urinary retention, see your internist, who may then refer you to an urologist.

Ultrasound can be used to see if there is urinary retention. The patient is asked to empty his bladder, and ultrasound is used to estimate how much urine remains. This is called a "post void residual."

In the "Infection" chapter, we discussed the effect of a urinary-tract infection on the elderly. Confusion is often the only symptom. Sometimes weakness is prominent and can result in a fall. If a normally independent elderly person suddenly has difficulty taking care of him or herself, a urinary-tract infection should be considered as the primary cause.

If your pet dog starts acting "run down," urinating frequently, and has a warm nose/fever, watch the urine. If the urine is cloudy or bad smelling, a course of antibiotics will probably fix the dog right up. It sure has worked for our female dogs over the years!

It is interesting to note that it is challenging to diagnose a young child with a UTI, and then it becomes hard again when a person is over sixty years old. Ah, the cycle of life! In both the child and the elderly person, a change in behavior, whether or not accompanied by a fever, should prompt a test of the urine.

Sometime a "urine dip" is enough to make the diagnosis. Most ERs have test strips, and it only takes a minute to have the answer. If there is no history of recurrent infection, and if there are no complicating factors, such as diabetes, this may be a reasonable approach.

If the urine goes to the lab and is found to be infected, it will generally be designated for a "culture and sensitivity." The culture attempts to determine if there is a "dominant organism." The urine specimen, even with a clean catch, is not sterile, but an infection will be caused by a certain type of bacteria that is out of control. If a bunch of different bacteria normally found in the body grow with equal speed and number, the urine is considered normal and not infected. The dominant bacterium (the cause of the infection) is grown by the lab and then tested for sensitivity to different antibiotics. The whole process takes two to three days. If the antibiotic you are given is not the right one for your infection, you should be called and a new antibiotic prescribed. Be sure you give a good phone number!

Some urinary tract infections cause a lot of blood in the urine, which is known as hemorrhagic cystitis. "Hematuria" is the medical word for blood in the urine. If you have hematuria, an infection may be the problem, but if the blood does not go away, bladder cancer and other problems must be considered.

Kidney Stones

Kidney stones are a major problem for some people, and others will never be so unfortunate. A kidney stone is a hard piece of "gravel," usually made of calcium. Kidney stones can vary in size from barely visible (or smaller) to filling the entire kidney. The big ones that fill the kidney are known as "staghorn calculi" because they develop a pronged shape, conforming to the multiple kidney ducts.

The stones that cause the most pain are the ones in the range of two to 10 millimeters in size. These tend to break off from the kidney and head down the ureter toward the bladder. As they move down the ureter, they cause a cramping, severe, knifelike pain that at first starts in the kidney area (flank) and moves downward, often radiating around toward the bladder. Men often describe the pain as going toward the testicles. As the ureter contracts to move the urine along, the pain increases, and when it relaxes, the pain decreases. This fluctuating pain is known as "renal colic." Most people who are passing their first kidney stone say it is the worst pain they have ever felt, though some say a low-back spasm is worse. Women who have delivered babies are mixed in their opinions. Some rank kidney-stone pain higher, and others give the pain of delivery the nod. The pain of passing a kidney stone decreases greatly as soon as it drops from the narrow tube of the ureter into the bladder. In most cases only a mild discomfort then remains.

A CT scan, if one is done, may show other stones in the kidneys. If these are still in the kidney, they do not cause pain. It is when they start their journey toward the bladder that the pain starts.

Sudden onset of a sharp pain in the flank radiating around to the front, with blood in the urine, whether visible or microscopic, is typical of a stone. Sometimes the patient's description of the pain, combined with a history of having had stones before, and now a test showing blood in the urine is enough for the physician to make the diagnosis. It is often hard for a person passing a stone to make urine. There is no clear reason for this, since even if the stone is completely obstructing one side, there is still a normal kidney working. This difficulty making urine probably has to do with the effect of pain and nerve stimulation. It is hard to urinate when tense, and the severe pain of a kidney stone certainly causes a person to be tense.

The big difference between a kidney stone and other causes of severe abdominal pain is that with a kidney stone there is either no abdominal tenderness or very little tenderness. Also, the person passing a kidney stone does not experience an increase in pain with movement. Writhing is common as the person tries unsuccessfully to find a position of comfort. People with most of the other causes of severe abdominal pain, such as appendicitis, experience increased pain with movement. A person with appendicitis will lie still in bed and move only reluctantly. When I push on the abdomen of someone who is passing a kidney stone, there is generally no change in the pain. Sometimes I need to ask the question, "Does pushing on your abdomen make the pain worse?" The person is in such discomfort that I am not able to tell if palpation has made a change. The answer is usually something along the lines of, "It hurts bad…mashing on my abdomen didn't make it much worse."

Seeing the stone on X-ray or CT is not needed right away if the person has a history of stones. Good pain control is needed, and the person can be sent home with more pain medication. Avoiding CT scans, with their substantial radiation dose, if not absolutely required is a good idea. Ultrasound can often be used to confirm the presence of a stone, and can help minimize radiation exposure. If the pain continues for more than a few days, a CT scan/ultrasound or other test will probably be needed to see the location of the stone and determine if it will pass on its own. Stones smaller than five millimeters will usually pass, and those larger than five millimeters often will not. If a stone is not making progress, referral to a urologist will be needed. The urologist can either recommend a process called lithotripsy, which breaks up the stone with focused shock/sound waves, or retrieve the stone via the bladder with a scope. Neither of these processes is completely painless, so if the stone will pass on its own, let it.

The kidney can handle complete obstruction, with no urine flow, for at least a week without suffering damage. For the kidney it is like being "on vacation." The blood flow continues, but the work is on hold. Eventually the kidney will suffer damage, though, so remaining in touch with the urologist while the stone is passing is vital.

If you have kidney stones, it is important to have one analyzed. You will be given a strainer to catch the stone and a bottle so you can take it to your doctor. Though calcium oxalate stones are the commonest, there are other types as well. There are things to do to decrease the chance of more stones, and these vary, depending on the type of stone. Drinking more water on a daily basis is a good place to start. If you are a coffee drinker, making your coffee with distilled water might help even more. This is especially true if your water is very high in minerals. Adding several glasses of distilled water will not only improve your hydration while decreasing the amount of minerals that form stones in the kidney, it will make the coffee taste better!

Renal (kidney) function is measured by using two tests that we discussed in "The Medical Laboratory" chapter: creatinine (Cr) and blood urea nitrogen (BUN). These are two waste products that the kidneys remove. Dehydration will cause both of these to rise. The BUN will rise more than the Cr if dehydration/decreased blood volume is the cause of the failure. The kidneys cannot do their job if they aren't filtering/cleaning as much blood. If the level of creatinine starts to rise in a consistent manner, there is a problem with renal function. Since a person can donate a kidney without a rise in BUN/ Cr, apparently the total kidney function must drop to less than half for these levels to rise. Nephrology is the specialty that addresses the medical aspects of kidneys. The nephrologists or internists will be charged with discovering the reason for the decreased function.

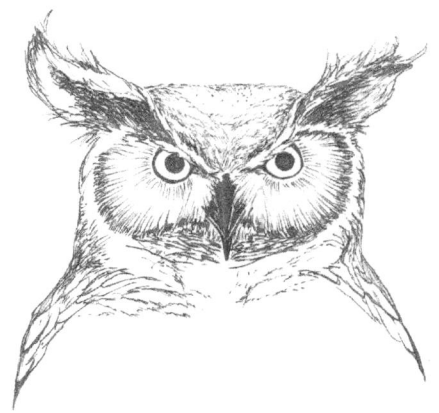

Chapter 42
Weakness

If you think a weakness can be turned into a strength, I hate to tell you this, but that's another weakness.

—*Jack Handy*

Denial ain't just a river in Egypt.

—*Mark Twain*

The causes of weakness are multiple and diverse. As a matter of fact, a good computer diagnostic program can list nearly five hundred causes of weakness! In this chapter we will not attempt to discuss all five hundred causes, but instead we will go over the basic concepts

These concepts will allow you narrow the range of possibilities and probably either come up with the answer or help your doctor do so. We will also discuss some of the commoner causes in more detail.

When someone complains of weakness, the first thing to determine is whether this is a "weak-all-over" sort of weakness or a "my arm won't move" sort of weakness. In medicine we say generalized weakness versus focal weakness. If the weakness is focal, involving a specific part of the body or side of the body, the cause is usually structural.

Stroke

A stroke, known medically as a cerebrovascular accident (CVA), causes the relatively sudden loss of the ability to move or feel a part of the body. Strokes can also cause loss of vision, and this is usually partial, but often involves parts of the visual field of both eyes. A stroke can cause loss of or alteration in thought processes and speech, as well. We discussed the bleeding type of stroke in the "Headache" chapter. Bleeding of the brain accounts for about 10 percent of strokes. The other 90 percent are caused by cessation of blood flow to a section of the brain. The symptoms are related to that particular section. The left side of the brain controls the right side of the body, and the right side controls the left. Thus a stroke of the left brain (motor cortex) causes a loss of movement of the right side of the body.

The nonbleeding strokes are thought to be caused by blood clotting. Either a small clot forms in the heart—possibly as a result of an arrhythmia such as atrial fibrillation (see "Shortness of Breath" chapter)—and breaks off, moving up the carotid artery to the brain and blocking flow to an area, or a narrowed part of the carotid artery itself is obstructed. These strokes do not cause headache initially. Weakness of an arm and the leg on the same side, as well as facial weakness and possibly voice change, are typical of a serious stroke.

Chapter 42 Weakness

Sometimes the symptoms of a stroke will appear but then go away, leaving no change. This is called a transient ischemic attack, or TIA. A TIA should not be ignored and deserves a thorough and prompt investigation. A permanent stroke follows the TIA in a large percent of cases, and the TIA should be considered a lucky warning in the same way that anginal chest pain can be a warning that a heart attack may be coming.

After a TIA, the carotid arteries need to be examined with ultrasound to see if there is narrowing. The heart needs to be checked for arrhythmia, both with an EKG and by monitoring. Magnetic resonance imaging is assuming a larger role in stroke diagnosis, and asking about an MRI is a good idea. CT is still the initial imaging study of choice since it is faster and often more readily available. The primary utility of the CT scan is to quickly differentiate between bleeding and clotting strokes.

It is easy for elderly people to deny that they are having a stroke. Aha—that denial problem rears its ugly head again! Many elderly people fear strokes and think about them a lot. I don't blame them for worrying. Ignoring the symptoms of a stroke, though, won't make it go away. If the symptoms are serious, and if the patient gets to the ER soon enough, some clot-dissolving medications can be given. After four hours or so, these medications are not as useful, and since they can cause bleeding, they are not given if the person arrives too late.

The history of the weakness is important. Did it come on suddenly or slowly? Was something eaten recently that was suspect, such as old canned food? Has there been illness or dehydration? Is there a family history of problems causing weakness?

Weakness can be either true weakness or perceived weakness. When I conduct my physical exam to diagnose the cause of weakness, I will have the person perform many maneuvers. Some of these, such as standing on the toes of one foot, are tests of both strength and balance. Some, such as squeezing my fingers, test strength. There are repetitive movements designed to test endurance of a particular muscle group. Sometimes a muscle will start out weak, but then get stronger with repetition.

If the weakness involves a part of the arm or leg, but not the whole arm or leg, for example, a smaller nerve of the arm or leg might be the cause of the weakness. We talked about carpal tunnel syndrome in the "Extremity Pain without Trauma" chapter. If the carpal tunnel compresses the median nerve, weakness of the muscles that oppose the thumb and forefinger can result. Likewise, if the ulnar nerve ("funny bone") is compressed at the elbow, numbness of the fifth finger is experienced, and weakness and atrophy of the muscles that move the fingers apart and together can occur.

Back pain of the sciatic variety can be accompanied by weakness. If this occurs, the weakness is of the muscle that lifts the foot off the ground (difficulty standing on the heels). Snagging/stubbing the toe on the ground repeatedly while walking may be the first symptom. This is called "foot drop" and should result in an immediate MRI to diagnose the cause. Compression of the sacral nerves can cause loss of control of the bowel or bladder. This is a serious problem that demands immediate diagnosis and treatment, as well.

Electrolyte imbalances and dehydration can cause weakness. Low potassium is typical in this regard, though mildly low potassium is not usually noticed. Low sodium is more often a cause of confusion and disorientation than a cause of weakness. A low blood sugar can cause weakness, as can a high blood sugar.

Diarrhea can cause weakness both by lowering the potassium and by causing dehydration.

Botulism is an interesting and unique cause of weakness. *Clostridium botulinum* is a bacterium that produces a toxin that causes muscular paralysis. Honey acts as a reservoir for the bacteria, and infants less than a year old are susceptible to having these spores multiply in their intestinal tract and produce toxin. Thus, honey is not recommended for children less than a year old. Over 90 percent of food botulism cases occur to children under the age of six months. After that time, the intestines are thoroughly colonized by bacteria, and there is no room for the bad bacteria to set up shop.

Adults exposed to the toxin can suffer paralysis as well. *Clostridium botulinum* is an anaerobic bacterium and thus can live in a sealed can. If the can is opened and the contents eaten without adequate cooking, poisoning can result. Boiling at sea level will destroy the toxin, but may not destroy the bacteria. The contaminated food will thus be safe for adults after boiling for more than a few minutes, but possibly not safe for infants. Botulism is also occasionally seen after injections associated with drug abuse. A large series of these cases occurred while I was a resident rotating in the intensive care unit at University of California Davis. Though ventilator support is often needed, the majority of people with botulism survive.

Weakness can be caused by either cardiac or pulmonary problems. The heart is like the body's motor, and if its "horsepower" decreases, almost everything else suffers. Usually this will not be a weakness of maximal strength in the short term, but rather of endurance in the short term and both strength and endurance in the long term. Shortness of breath is usually present.

A Sad Case of Cardiac Weakness and Denial

One of the saddest cases of weakness with a cardiac cause that I have ever treated involved a fourteen-year-old boy. I was working in a small ED at the time, shortly after residency, and we had twelve-hour shifts. I was working five day- shifts in a row. The first time I saw Nate was after he ate lunch at school. He vomited most of what he ate, and since he had vomited after lunch on the previous day also, his mother brought him in. He had no medical history and had only seen the pediatrician for required checkups. He was a bit pale, but otherwise his exam and vital signs were normal. He pinked up after some nausea medicine and fluids by mouth, and I sent him home improved.

His parents brought him back the next day at about the same time. Once again he had nausea and vomiting. An unwritten rule in emergency medicine is. "When a patient returns, always go at least one step farther." I did note that he was pale on the previous visit, so I ordered an IV and some fluid, sending blood to the lab. The blood count (CBC) and chemistry (see "The Medical Laboratory" chapter) were normal. He looked better after the fluid and antiemetic. Despite his pallor, there was no anemia. Once again I sent him home improved.

On the third day, his parents brought him back again. Once again he was vomiting after eating. About the only things I hadn't already checked were a chest X-ray and EKG. I ordered these, along with a few esoteric labs very unlikely to be useful in a four-teen-year-old. The chest X-ray showed a hugely dilated heart! On further detailed questioning, he had been experiencing a slow pro-gression of symptoms over the last six months or so, culminat-ing in decreased blood flow to the intestines and food intolerance. When I began to ask probing questions, it developed that he had stopped participating in sports six months earlier because "they just weren't fun anymore." He had experienced increasing weak-ness and shortness of breath with exertion and thus "just didn't do hard stuff anymore."

Our cardiologist came to see him, and after a series of tests, he was determined to have "myocarditis and dilated cardiomyopathy, most likely secondary to a combination of the common cold and bad luck." The cardiologist explained that while CHF (congestive heart failure) in the elderly causes typical symptoms (see "Shortness of Breath" chapter), in children it often affects the bowel first. We discussed how in CHF fluid enters the lungs. Well, it also causes swelling of the wall of the stomach and bowel, which results in food intolerance.

Nate was put on the transplant list. Unfortunately a good donor match was not easily found, and he came to the ER many times as the months passed. Each time the parents acted as if they had no clue as to why he was vomiting! They had the strongest ability to deny disease that I had ever witnessed. Nate was an only child, and they just absolutely refused to believe he was in serious trouble. Even after numerous meetings with the cardiologist, and my repeated detailed explanations, they still refused to believe he had a problem. It came, over the months, to the point where I tried speaking loudly, and invoked my social worker and all of her powers of persuasion. I remember at one point saying; "You should be camping on the steps at Stanford!" The parents continued to fail to actually believe that there was a problem. He looked worse and worse, despite all the miracles modern medicine could do, and eventually died. This was a devastating blow to his parents, though initially they seemed to not be surprised. Even after he died, they did not accept and understand what had happened. Over the course of the next 3 months they both internalized the whole experience. Two months later the father arrived in a state of complete emotional collapse, and required hospitalization in our psychiatric unit. Three months after Nate's death his mother attempted suicide, and was hospitalized as well. Denial was not the answer, but neither was belated acceptance.

When a young athletic person who doesn't understand medicine brags that he or she has a "large heart," I try to smile and nod, but inside I feel a bit of pain and hope they are mistaken. A "normal" sized heart is what you want—take my word for it. An athlete's heart may be very slightly larger, slightly stronger, and more efficient, but it should not be noticeably bigger, and the muscle should not be much, if at all, thicker. If the heart becomes noticeably larger, it is time to see the cardiologist for some testing. Just look at that marathon runner's legs. Are they noticeably enlarged? No, but they are toned and highly efficient. It is the same way with the athletic heart. Normal changes to an athlete's heart are quite subtle.

When an older person is weak, they may require additional help. Diagnosing a weak eighty-year-old with a urinary-tract infection implies that they will need help for at least a few days while they recover, if not an admission to the hospital. Falls are common during the recovery period and should be guarded against.

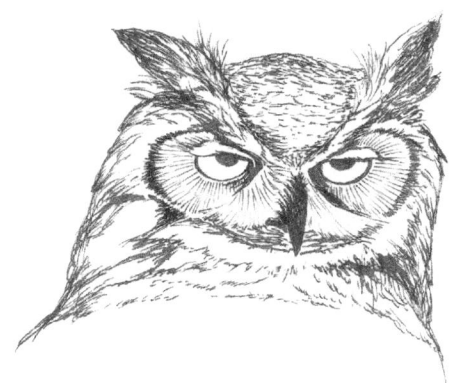

Chapter 43
Wounds and Wound Repair

*The United States lost more men from battle wounds and disease
in the Civil War than in any other war of its history, including the
Second World War. The battlefront stretched from Pennsylvania to
New Mexico, and included also the seven seas.*

—Ann Donovan

We talked about wounds in some detail in the "Bites and Stings"
chapter and about infection, which is a big part of wound care, in the
"Infection" chapter. By now you know quite a bit about infection and
will probably anticipate some of the information in this chapter.

Lacerations that need stitches are a common reason to visit the emergency department. Sometimes I won't repair a wound during a shift, but more often I will suture at least several before the day is through. On wound-prone days, I have done more than a dozen.

To Suture, or Not to Suture

The first decision to be made about a wound is whether it needs to be sutured (closed). Many factors are at play in answering this question. A wound to the arms or legs that is more than eight hours old will usually not be sutured. An older wound is more heavily contaminated and thus at a greater risk of infection. Facial wounds can go longer and will be closed (after cleansing, of course) out to and beyond twenty-four hours. The face has better circulation and is thus less likely to become infected. The cosmetic result is also very important in facial wounds and less so on the extremities.

Most people who come to the ER with a laceration don't realize that any time a wound is sutured, there is increased risk of serious infection. We touched upon this principle in the "Bites and Stings" chapter. Even a large wound, if left open, will generally heal just fine, though it will take longer and result in a bigger scar.

A skillful wound closure will decrease scarring, speed healing, and give a very satisfying and cosmetically superior result. The first skill involved in skillful wound closure is deciding if the wound should be closed.

Natural Wound Healing

In 1996 a college student found a skeleton on the shore of the Columbia River. The remains were examined, and dating found them to be a bit over nine thousand years old. "Kennewick Man" had led a rough life. He had evidence of multiple rib fractures. A stone spearpoint was lodged in his pelvis. He had suffered serious head injury, which very likely caused a substantial laceration. It is estimated that he was between forty and fifty years old when he died. His wounds were old, with signs of healing, and not the apparent cause of his death.

When the Kennewick Man suffered a laceration, he almost certainly did not expect it to be sutured. Most likely the wound was covered to some extent and allowed to dry. If there was obvious foreign material, such as sticks and pieces of dirt in the wound, it was likely removed. The dirt that remained would be included in the blood clot that filled and covered the wound (scab). When the itching started, the Kennewick Man would likely scratch at the scab, and it would come off, carrying with it most of the dirt that was in the wound. Meanwhile, the wound was healing from the inside, and the body was forcing contaminants such as dirt and gravel to the surface, where they could be removed with the next scab. Eventually, the wound would become smaller and smaller. An itchy, pink scar would then remain. Eventually, it would stop itching.

When I was growing up, children cared for their wounds in this way. The nasty scabs that I had on my knees from skateboard crashes had to come off a time or two before those deep abrasions would heal all the way. I remember seeing gravel imbedded in a scab that a fellow skateboarder showed me.

If Kennewick Man walked to the nearest "Medicine Man" with his dirty wound, and it was cleaned very thoroughly and sutured, one of two things would happen after he walked back down to the river. If it was indeed the type of wound that can be cleaned well enough to suture—in other words, not a puncture, recent enough, and not badly contaminated—he might do very well, with less scarring and faster healing than if he had left the wound open. If there was a bit of dirt deep in a recess of the wound that the Medicine Man did not see and remove, he would then be in serious trouble. With the wound sutured shut, his body could not easily get rid of that dirt. Pus would accumulate around the dirt. Probably it would more easily move between the deeper tissue layers than escape to the surface. The unfortunate

Kennewick Man would likely make it to a cave as the pain increased. Fever would set in as the infection reached the lymph nodes, and shaking chills would begin as the infection entered his bloodstream. His deep infection would be very difficult, if not impossible, for him to survive.

If his spear wound (with the embedded spear point) had been sutured, I guarantee his skeleton would not have shown signs of healing! Here's why. Any visible amount of contamination in a wound guarantees an infection. Any visible foreign material must be removed before the wound can be sutured. Removal of the dirt is known as "debridement." Blunt debridement might be scrubbing or grabbing with tweezers, and sharp debridement is cutting out badly damaged and thoroughly contaminated tissue with a scalpel or sharp scissor.

Leaving anything organic (made by a living creature, whether animal or plant) in the wound will essentially guarantee infection. This includes dirt, since dirt contains a lot of organic material. All such material must be removed before wound closure. The bacterial counts are too high for the body's immune system to overcome.

I often talk to hikers and hunters who would like to learn how to suture. I will explain the methods in good detail below, so you will have a leg up if you need to do so; however, the best bet will almost always be to leave the wound open and concentrate on control of bleeding, cleansing, and good dressings. The risk of infection in wounds sutured in the field is just too high. Even if the infection is not life threatening, a wound infection causes increased scarring and loss of function and should not be risked.

Every wound that comes to the ER is contaminated to some degree. What matters is the degree. If the bacterial count is low enough, the body can conquer/destroy the bacteria before they get out of control. If there are too many to conquer initially, the battle must be fought, and we call that battle "infection."

Chapter 43 Wounds and Wound Repair

Materials such as glass and metal (such as a bullet) are less porous and have a lower number of bacteria. There is a probability that these will cause an infection, however, because they will become surrounded by a blood clot, which allows bacteria to multiply before the body can send in the troops we talked about in the "Infection" chapter. Glass and metal can sometimes cause a low-grade infection rather than the nasty aggressive type caused by wood, dirt, cloth, or other organic material. Some porous material can be drawn into the wound with the non porous object, such as in the case of a low velocity bullet, and this porous material will cause infection if not removed. Sometimes the body will clean up a metal or glass foreign body and reach a "peaceful truce," wherein the foreign body can remain in the body for the rest of the person's life. Often, though, the truce will be temporary, and a bullet or piece of glass will be rejected and emerge months or years later. I have, so far, removed four bullets that had been embedded for over a year. One had been in place since the Vietnam War! I rallied my "troops" and that gent must have shaken at least 50 hands before leaving the ED that day.

A nice clean knife wound or glass cut that comes to the ER promptly and is larger than one centimeter will most likely be sutured after cleansing, and the result will probably be very nice.

Local Anesthetic and Nerve Blocks

Before the wound is irrigated, and certainly before it is sutured, the wound should be anesthetized. Local anesthetics such as lidocaine, and the longer lasting marcaine/sensorcaine, are standard. These solutions come either with or without epinephrine. We mentioned epinephrine (adrenaline) in the "Bites and Stings" chapter and several other places. In wound anesthesia, epinephrine is used to tighten up the blood vessels around the wound, which slows bleeding. Epinephrine is generally not used on fingertips, earlobes, and other places where decreasing the circulation isolates a body part, though the risk of doing so is likely overestimated. Epinephrine is especially good on scalp and some facial wounds that tend to bleed a lot. Local anesthetics sting a bit and feel like getting lemon juice into the wound. Fortunately, the sting only lasts for a few seconds before numbness sets in. It is much less painful if the anesthetic is injected through the cut edge of the wound, rather than making new skin punctures, and it should be injected into the soft tissue beneath the skin, rather than into the tough, dense skin itself. There are far fewer sensitive nerve endings beneath the skin than in the skin layers, and the tissue beneath the skin can more easily stretch to accept the anesthetic. This injection of the anesthetic directly into the wound edges is known as "infiltration."

Another good way to anesthetize a wound is by using regional anesthesia. Regional anesthesia is one of the areas of emergency medicine I have continued to teach since leaving UC Davis. A wound can sometimes be completely anesthetized with a single and relatively painless injection near the nerve that serves the area of the wound, rather than by injecting into the wound itself. Every emergency physician has some knowledge of nerve blocks, though the level of knowledge varies from physician to physician. Asking your doctor if a nerve block can be used for pain control is worthwhile.

Nerve blocks can ease pain in other injuries and painful conditions, as well as in wounds. Remember the "Dental Pain" chapter? Other pain often responds just as well to a nerve block as does a toothache. When we discussed knee replacement in the "Extremity Pain without Trauma" chapter, we went over regional anesthetic options for knee replacement. Many surgeries can be performed with nerve blocks, thus avoiding the risks of general anesthesia. If your emergency physician is not familiar with the particular nerve block needed to anesthetize your injury, he or she can review using a procedural text or receive instruction on my website.

The most frequently needed nerve block in the ER for wound repair is the "digital nerve block." Performing a digital nerve block is simple, and every emergency physician knows the procedure. Several milliliters of lidocaine or other local anesthetic (without epinephrine) is injected through a very thin, short needle into the base of the finger. Two injections are usually needed, one on each side of the finger. The nerves that bring the pain and sensation from the finger to the hand are thus "blocked," and feeling to the finger is interrupted. If you have a digital nerve block for a finger laceration, you will still feel the finger when it is pulled on or bumped, because it is still attached to your body. I usually demonstrate the difference in feeling to the patient by tugging on their pant leg. When I tug on the pant leg or shirt sleeve, they feel it, but it doesn't hurt. Tugging on the numb finger—which should be just as numb as the pant leg or shirt sleeve after a successful nerve block—will still be felt, but only because it is attached to a body part that still has sensation.

Cleansing and Debridement

After the wound is anesthetized, it should be thoroughly cleansed. The amount of cleansing needed varies according to the condition of the wound, of course. If there is visible dirt and contamination, it must all be removed. High-pressure irrigation is the standard method. Dribbling some saline into the wound is not good enough, and if you watch, you will see that dribbling does not remove any of the visible dirt. Hard squirting is required. Special adapters are available to prevent a lot of splashing and to focus the stream so it is strong enough. You should hear a "SHHHH" sound as the fluid hits the wound.

Scrubbing may also be needed to get the wound clean, and there are special scrub brushes with cleanser made for the purpose. Every part of the wound must be seen, examined, and cleaned. Most wounds have some blood-clot adhering, and that must be broken loose before irrigation. Irrigation alone will not break the blood clot loose to expose the entire wound; this usually needs to be done with either the catheter or a metal instrument such as a hemostat. Nurses and techs do most of the irrigation of wounds. I usually anesthetize the wound and then complete the discharge paperwork while the wound is irrigated/cleaned by one of my techs. There is a great tendency for the nurse or tech to be gentle with the wound. They are caring and empathetic people who do not like to risk inflicting pain. The wound is numb, however, and this is no time for gentleness.

When I return to the cleansed wound, my first step is exploration. I explore the wound to look for damage to deep structures, including bones, tendons, joints, and nerves, and to ensure that I know the extent of the wound. I also ensure that the entire wound has been cleansed. If a section was missed, I will scrub or irrigate as needed to ensure the entire wound is free of visible contamination.

At this stage I also will debride, as we discussed above, as needed. There are often pieces of yellow or white globules of fat in the wound that are contaminated, and I will remove these. The pieces of fat are not needed, and since they have less circulation than the rest of the wound, are likely to act as a source of infection. Any hairs must be removed, and though shaving is rarely needed, antibiotic ointment is sometimes helpful to "slick back" hair from a scalp wound. Sometimes a scissor can be used to shorten the hair at the wound edge. Shaving is not usually recommended since it generates lots of small bits of hair, which are hard to reliably remove from the wound, and hair is far from sterile.

The next step is suturing. Sutures fall into two basic categories: absorbable and nonabsorbable. Within these categories there are various thicknesses and needle sizes. In the emergency department, absorbable suture is used less frequently than in the operating room. Most surgical incisions are sterile, and a buried absorbable suture usually does not cause a problem. Few, if any, of our wounds in the ER are sterile, and therefore buried, absorbable sutures serve as a starting point for infection. A bit of clot will surround each suture, and the body will have a harder time penetrating that clot to "clear up" the bacteria during the healing process.

Sometimes absorbable suture is used in pediatric patients so they don't need to have their stitches removed. Pinning down a crying three-year-old to remove the sutures is tough, and I can see the temptation to use absorbable suture for skin closure. I usually do not, however, since absorbable suture is made to be buried and does not absorb well at the surface of the skin. The parent needs to be able to accept the strings that will be hanging out of their child for a few weeks as the downside of "absorbable" skin sutures.

When I worked in an ED where many of the doctors used absorbable suture on children, the following scenario was common: a parent would bring a child back a week or so after the wound was repaired and would complain that the sutures did not seem to be absorbing. I would try to remove the supposedly "absorbable" sutures for them. Absorbable suture is not slippery like the nonabsorbable one, and thus when cut will not pull easily out of the skin. The best bet was to use a small scissor to cut the sutures off close to the skin, to make "shorter stubble" out of them, rather than trying to pull them out.

Closing irregularly shaped wounds can be a challenge. The first step is to find a landmark, if one exists. Sometimes a wrinkle can be used to ensure proper alignment. With a V-shaped wound, the first stitch should be at the point of the V. This pins the flap down. If I were to start at one side of the V, I might get to the point of the V and find that it doesn't line up where it should. Alignment must be perfect, since a misaligned wound will scar badly. In the V-shaped laceration, the next two sutures will go at the midpoints of the "legs" of the V. If the wound is then nicely approximated, the job is done. If there are still gaps, the resulting spaces can be divided with more sutures. If you sketch it out, you will see that a V-shaped laceration with equal sides will require an odd number of sutures to be symmetrical.

Medical Wisdom

A linear laceration will usually receive the first suture in the middle, and the remaining halves will then be each divided with two more sutures. If the first suture is placed at one end of the wound rather than at the middle, unequal wound tensions will usually make it seem that one side of the wound is longer than the other when the end is reached, and the longer side will want to bunch up."This is called a "dog ear" and is an error that will result in scarring.

Note that I used the word "approximate" above. The rule in suturing is "approximate, don't strangulate." The wound edges should be brought together gently, with no additional force added. If the suture is too tight, it will cause blanching (turning white, rather than pink) at the wound edge. Blanching indicates that the blood flow to the wound edge is being reduced. If the suture is not loosened, the wound will not be able to heal at that point. The suture can be loosened by gently inserting the small and very pointy iris scissor into the suture after it is tied. The scissor is then opened, stretching the suture and tightening the knot from within the loop of suture. If the wound swells after you are sent home and you see blanching along the suture line, you can either loosen the suture yourself or return to have the wound rechecked.

Sometimes a "running suture" is used. In a running suture, a stitch is placed at one end, and the wound is sewed "clothing style" toward the other end and then secured. The upside of this technique is speed. The downsides are several. It is hard to loosen the sutures afterward as described above. I have removed quite a few tight running sutures over the years that looked all right when the patient came back. Unfortunately, the wound popped right open when the suture was removed! There had not been enough blood flow to the wound edge for healing. It is harder to customize the running wound closure by changing the angle, depth, and direction with each suture to achieve a perfect approximation. Fewer sutures are better in most cases, as long as a perfect approximation of edges results, and a running suture means the sutures must continue the length of the wound whether needed or not.

A wound that is gaping (under tension) requires pressure to bring it together, and that pressure must be distributed widely and gently. If there is a choice between taking "small bites" by inserting the needle close to the wound edge and "larger bites" by inserting the needle farther from the wound edge, taking a bigger bite is usually the right choice. The bigger bite spreads the pressure required to bring the edges together over a bigger area. Since there is less pressure per unit area, the blood is better able to reach the wound edge, and better healing occurs.

Wound glue and Steri-Strips or butterfly bandages can also be used to close wounds. If the wound is gaping, though, these methods do not work very well. Wound glue only works on dry skin, so the inside of the wound is still under tension. A blood clot below the skin's surface will form in the gap that results from that tension, and this will become a scar. Also, the glue will usually not resist the tension long enough for the wound to heal, and the wound will open.

The Steri-Strip/butterfly closure works well for the superficial, but sometimes large skin tears that are often seen in the elderly. Once approximated, these wounds generally have little or no tension and heal well. Wound glue works well on wounds that are self-approximating (not gaping), and glue may help keep the wound immobile and cleaner in that situation. Since there is no tension, and the wound is already approximated, it would also do fine if allowed to heal naturally. There is a stronger argument for using glue on self-approximating wounds in children than in adults, who are likelier to take good care of their wound.

Patients always ask, "How many stitches will I get?" My answer is, "Just enough to do a perfect job." Once the wound edges are brought together and the pressure spread evenly and gently, there is nothing to gain from more stitches.

Sometimes a dirty wound must be closed in an attempt to improve the cosmetic result, but the chance of infection must be reduced as well. In these cases, a "loose closure" is sometimes possible. In a loose closure, a perfect approximation is not attempted, since it would cause an unacceptable increase in the chance of infection. The wound is improved, however, and while it is allowed to drain (ooze/ weep as it cleans itself), a smaller scar should result. Another option is a "delayed primary closure." After four days or so of treatment by dressing changes only, the wound will either be displaying signs of surface infection, or it will be cleaner looking and brighter in color. At that time the wound may be able to be closed loosely.

Antibiotics?

Antibiotics should be discussed next. As we mentioned in the "Fractures and Dislocations" chapter, open fractures are generally treated with antibiotics. Bite wounds are also often treated with antibiotics. Most other fresh wounds do not need prophylactic antibiotics. Most wounds will not get infected if cared for properly. A wound that has organic foreign material in it—or any foreign material, for that matter—will get infected no matter how many antibiotics the patient takes. If a wound that is "teetering on the brink" of infection does get antibiotics and goes on to become infected anyway, there is a chance the infection will be resistant to antibiotics and therefore harder to treat. Since most wounds won't get infected, it is generally better to wait and then use antibiotics as needed. Elevating and immobilizing the injured part will speed healing and decrease the chance of infection. Elevating the extremity reduces swelling, which improves circulation. Splinting and an absorbent dressing prevents the "in and out" movement of fluids that can further contaminate the wound.

If a sutured wound does get infected, standard treatment is to remove the sutures, cleanse the wound, and leave it open, with dressing changes. The wound can then either be allowed to heal naturally, or a delayed closure can be done after the infection is gone.

Dressings

A dressing will be applied, or at least a Band-Aid, before you leave the ER. The primary purpose of a dressing is to absorb the drainage from the wound. By absorbing the drainage, more drainage is encouraged, which helps the body decrease the bacterial count cf the wound. Drainage that is absorbed also cannot repeatedly enter and exit the wound with movement. The dressing helps prevent the wound from sealing itself closed, as well, and helps to keep the wound clean and free of sunburn. The wound, whether sutured or not, will probably be coated with an antibiotic ointment such as Bacitracin or Neosporin before the dressing is placed. The antibiotic ointment helps in a number of ways: Wounds heal better when they are moist, and the ointment encourages moistness. The antibiotic also helps the dressing prevent the wound from drying and thus sealing itself before the drainage can escape.

The dressings also look good, especially when done by a skilled ER Tech!

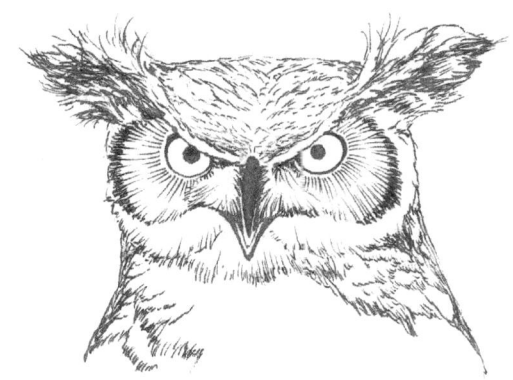

Chapter 44
X-Ray and Radiology

If the hand be held between the discharge tube and the screen,
the darker shadow of the bones is seen within the slightly dark
shadow-image of the hand itself...for brevity's sake I shall use the
expression "rays"; and to distinguish them from others of this
name I shall call them "X-rays."

—Wilhelm Conrad Rontgen

You have probably had an X-ray at some point. Whether this was a chest X-ray to look for pneumonia, or an ankle X-ray to see if that swollen ankle was broken, X-rays are a very commonly performed and useful test.

X-rays use radiation to penetrate the injured part and expose a sensitive plate placed behind it. The body varies in density, and bones are the densest. Therefore, where the bone is, the least X-ray energy will reach the other side, and the most will pass through where there is air, such as the lung on the chest X-ray. In other words, bone will stop the most X-ray energy, and air the least. The varying density of the different body tissues creates a picture that can then be interpreted. The intermediate density tissues, such as muscle, fat, tendons, and ligaments, are similar enough in density that it is hard to tell them apart on a plain X-ray. Magnetic resonance imaging (MRI), however, can easily distinguish among these different tissues when that is needed. Computed tomography (CT) also does a better job on tissue detail, though not nearly as good as the MRI.

Radiation Exposure

A standard X-ray does not result in very much radiation exposure. A chest X-ray, for example, is only equal to an average of ten days' exposure to the normal background radiation in our environment. In other words, everyone gets about forty X-rays worth of radiation a year if they never go to the doctor! Computed tomography is a different matter, however. A CT of the abdomen and pelvis with and without contrast material (we'll discuss contrast soon) equals about four hundred chest X-rays! That is ten years of environmental radiation exposure all at once. Obviously CT scans should be performed only when really needed.

To understand why a CT involves so much radiation, it helps to understand how a CT scanner works. CT scanners look like big donuts. The part of a patient to be imaged fits within the donut, and the mechanism inside spins around, taking X-rays from all angles. The computer then assembles all those individual X-rays into a series of images. The patient is moved into the donut in small increments. Each centimeter that the patient is moved creates a new image. The image is spoken of as a "slice." Each slice requires another barrage of X-rays.

The advantage of CT over X-ray becomes apparent when I mention the weakness of basic X-ray. Say you take a knife and slice an apple perfectly down the middle, dividing it into two equal halves. Now keep the two halves together. Rotate the apple so you cannot see that it has been cut at all. If you held it in that position and shot an X-ray front to back, the X-ray would show a perfect apple. Looking at the X-ray, there would be no way to tell the apple was cut. Possibly a seed would be split, which might show—but otherwise there is no way to tell. Now rotate the apple so the cut is facing right toward you, clearly seen. That is the X-ray view that is going to show the "apple fracture" best. Still, there is no distance between the two halves, so the fracture, which is a nondisplaced apple fracture (remember the "Fractures and Dislocations" chapter?), will not likely show very well at all. At best it will show as a thin, straight line between the two halves. Now rotate the apple so that the cut is no longer visible. Move the two halves apart, but keep them perfectly aligned. An X-ray now would still be normal. Even though there is distance between the two halves (displaced apple fracture), they are aligned so the fracture cannot be seen. Now turn the halves, still holding them apart, so that it is clear that there are two halves. An X-ray from that angle will clearly show a displaced fracture. Every other point of rotation will have a different chance of showing the fracture. CT avoids this problem by shooting pictures from all angles. Regular X-ray, which we often refer to as "plain film/s" partially overcomes this weakness by shooting from at least two different angles when looking for a fracture.

The real danger of radiation exposure, with the resultant cancer risk, comes if you have a problem that is likely to require, or beg for, repeated CT scans. An example is kidney stones. Kidney stones are a recurrent problem, and if a person gets a CT each time they go the ER with flank pain and hematuria (blood in the urine), they will end up getting a lot of radiation exposure. Sometimes an ED will not be able to get records for a patient they have not seen before, and it may be easier and faster to just get a CT scan. If you have kidney stones, you will have to be your own advocate in this regard. The CT scan can wait in most cases, as we discussed in the "Urinary Problems" chapter, and if the stone passes, will no longer be needed.

Another factor to consider is that CT scanners are big money makers for a medical facility. A CT scanner is not cheap to purchase, and once purchased, costs about the same whether it is used a lot, or rarely. A CT tech will always be on duty, and a radiologist will usually be present, or on call, to read CT scans. The facility definitely has an incentive to encourage imaging. Whether that incentive is passed down to the ordering physicians openly or in a more subtle manner depends on the policies and reimbursement structure of the facility and of the physician group.

Sometimes it is worth asking about lead (the dense, heavy metal that blocks X-rays) drapes that can be used to keep the radiation from affecting sensitive areas. For example, the thyroid gland in the neck can be protected during a head CT or jaw (mandible) series. There are always a bunch of these lead gowns and covers lying around in the X-ray suite, and the X-ray techs will not think you are "funny" if you ask for them. Rather, they will think you are intelligent for being cautious. You may even catch them glancing at the radiation exposure badges they all wear!

The younger the patient, the greater is the risk of cancer from radiation exposure. Children younger than a year old are at an especially high risk. Doctors are now much more aware of this danger than when I was in training. A common story is the toddler who falls and hits his/her head. Twenty years ago, CTs were done in this case with impunity. Now doctors take the time to discuss the risk and benefit carefully with the parents. If there was no loss of consciousness with the fall, if the child is now acting normally and walking well, and if there is no suspected skull fracture on exam, the child is not likely to benefit from a CT scan, and the radiation exposure can be avoided.

My third child, Drake, had a large head. His head, when measured at routine visits to the pediatrician, was always off the top of the growth chart. On each of his three well-child visits during his first year, his pediatrician tried to talk me into bringing him in for a head CT. I plainly refused. I asked, "What do you expect to find on CT in a completely healthy, completely normal child?" She could not come up with anything that made any sense at all, but very strongly recommended the CT. Now Drake's body has caught up, and apparently there is a good brain in there, since he won his first two chess tournaments! CT scans are not to be recommended for children without good cause.

Magnetic resonance imaging does not cause radiation exposure. Before you have one, though, you will be asked a lot of questions. Ferrous metals (anything attracted to a magnet) cannot get near the very powerful magnetic attraction of the MRI scanner. There will be questions about claustrophobia as well, since an MRI scanner is a much smaller "donut" than the CT. If you are afraid of tight places, there are some medications that can help, such as Ativan or Valium. If you can tolerate caving (spelunking), you can tolerate an MRI without a problem.

A fluoroscope is an X-ray machine operated during a procedure, usually by stepping on a pedal. A screen is facing the operator, and an image is instantly available. I will use fluoroscopy occasionally when reducing (restoring to normal position) a displaced fracture. Nuclear medicine and radiologic procedures involving fluoroscopy can have a fairly high dose of radiation, but they are often very effective procedures that can substitute for surgery and therefore often worth every bit of it.

Contrast media is a dense liquid that resists X-ray penetration and therefore looks bright white on an X-ray. Contrast is given to highlight features and allow structures of similar density to be identifiable as separate. Contrast itself is not radioactive, but it can cause allergic reactions at times, especially the intravenous varieties. The intravenous varieties can also cause transient (goes away with time) renal failure. In the "Abdominal Pain" chapter, we discussed an X-ray called a barium contrast enema. Normally, a plain X-ray of the lower abdomen only shows the large bowel as a hazy structure with some dark patches of air and some slightly lighter areas of bowel contents, which is denser. If barium is given rectally, it spreads throughout the large bowel within minutes, outlining its every detail. The large bowel (colon) then looks bright white on the X-ray, appearing denser than, and thus blocking the view of, the spine. The detail seen on a barium enema completely dispels the myth that the colon is "full of toxic waste."

Ultrasound

Ultrasound has, over the last fifteen years, been widely adopted by emergency physicians. It is now safe to say that many of the very best clinical ultrasonographers are emergency physicians. Ultrasound is fast, portable, and carries no risk of radiation. An image is created by sending sound waves, and recording how they bounce back. Most well-equipped boats have one, but it is called a "depth sounder" or "fish finder"! Since I am a very enthusiastic fisherman, I immediately fell in love with ultrasound when it became available in the ER back in the early 1990s.

There are two ways of receiving an ultrasound in the ED. If the emergency physician brings the machine to your bedside, it is likely to answer a particular question. I used it yesterday, for example, to evaluate the fluid status of an extremely ill patient. Though young, the patient had a history of intravenous drug abuse and came in very short of breath with a high fever "for ten days." The portable chest X-ray looked like it could be either a bilateral pneumonia or congestive heart failure (CHF). It was likely the patient would be dehydrated, with the high fever and such severe shortness of breath, but he had very swollen feet and lower legs, with "pitting edema," a sign of fluid overload (see "Shortness of Breath" chapter).

Chapter 44 X-Ray and Radiology

I used the ultrasound to look at his vena cava. The vena cava (biggest vein) is a large, easily distended vein that runs through the abdomen to the heart. In CHF the vena cava should be distended, as the blood volume is increased. In dehydration it would be smaller and typically would collapse and refill with breathing. The vena cava was distended, with plenty of fluid reserve. In just a few seconds, I had determined that the man was volume loaded, rather than dehydrated.

Curiosity got the best of me, and I took a quick look at the heart. Though a formal echocardiogram would be needed to carefully examine the heart, I clearly saw that something was wrong with one of his heart valves. I also noted that the young heart was working very hard. In an intravenous drug abuser, infection of a heart valve (endocarditis) is a risk, and given his fever, that was almost certainly his problem. I slowed the fluids and loaded the patient with antibiotics. Ultrasound in the hands of a trained emergency physician is a very potent tool indeed.

The other type of ultrasound is a formal study. There is no substitute for a formal ultrasound when thorough evaluation is needed. I will order the ultrasound, and a professional ultrasonographer will perform the study and send it to the radiologist for interpretation. I always try to corner the ultrasonographer to get their impression as well, as what could be better?

Most X-ray tests you receive in large ERs will be ordered by the physician, performed by a technologist, and interpreted by another physician, the radiologist. Sometimes there is a delay in getting an X-ray interpretation by the radiologist, and often you will be sent home before it is available. If the radiologist does not agree with the emergency physician, you will be contacted and notified of the change. Results are also usually sent to your own doctor. If you will be seeing another doctor about the injury, it is a good idea to request the x-rays on Compact Disc. This was not possible just a few years ago, but can now be done in many facilities.

Conclusion

I hope this book has been helpful to you and that it will continue to be helpful. The world of medicine is changing rapidly. As I type this conclusion (after the fourth review) I am approaching five years since I wrote the first words of *Medical Wisdom*. Things have changed significantly already. Doctors continue to be under pressure to decrease costs; midlevel providers are being used more and more frequently in ERs. The government is working hard to restrict and manage medical care.

The Internet is a huge repository of data. There is an immense amount of medical information available. Much of this information is good and helpful, but there is a lot of misleading and false data, as well. It is even more important now that a person have both knowledge and "medical wisdom."

I would deeply appreciate input and plan to incorporate suggestions for additional content into the next edition. If there is a subject you would like covered, or a topic you feel should be expanded upon, please write me at my family website; www.windroseenterprises.com

For medical consultation, and to see an innovative new organization that specializes in patient advocacy and empowerment visit; www.MedicalNetworkUS.com

Additional copies of "Medical Wisdom" are available via both web-sites.

Mark Borden, MD, FAAEM
Emergency Physician

Epilogue

As more and more physicians have difficulty being paid for their services, more are becoming hospital employees. There are major downsides to the physician-employment model. Once physicians are employed, they are very subject to the "business and politics of medicine." When faced with demands to increase testing, or increase procedures an independent physician can say; "NO!" An employed physician, however can only say; "yes sir."

Each month at most hospitals, there is a meeting of the medical staff. In past years at that meeting, the doctors discussed important issues that had to do with patient care. Any time the business side (administration) made some decisions that seemed contrary to the best interests of their patients, doctors would discuss how to ensure that the patients, whom they care so much about, did not suffer. One point of leverage that doctors had was the referral. If a doctor chose, he could refer his patients to another hospital, and care for them there. This fact encouraged a hospital's administration to listen to the wishes of their doctors. Now that most of the doctors are employed by the hospital, they can no longer stand up to their hospital's administration and advocate for their patients. As a patient you may not be aware of this change in the model of physician practice, but you will definitely experience the difference!

Although emergency physicians are not employed by a hospital per se, they are employed by or are a member of a group that is employed by or contracted to provide services for a hospital. In this way they are under pressure to behave as the hospital administration wants them to.

One example I recently witnessed occurred when a hospital CEO decided that not enough CT scans were being ordered from his emergency department. This story demonstrates how pressure can be placed on a physician by a hospital. Remember from the "X-Ray and Radiology" chapter that a CT scan carries with it the downside of subjecting a patient to a lot of radiation—250 to 500 X-rays, sometimes even more. Physicians know that radiation should be avoided as often as possible.

The hospital administrator took a very simple business-management action. He decided to offer an incentive that encouraged physicians to order more CT scans. This worked to change the practice of several of the doctors. I am not saying these were bad doctors. One doctor in fact was heard to say, "Often the question of whether a CT is needed or not is unclear, and if ordering one results in a twenty-five-dollar bonus, then…what the heck!"

The CEO next decided to subject to review those physicians who ordered fewer than the average number of CT scans. Being reviewed is time consuming, stressful, and insulting. Some reviews also act as a black mark on a physician's record, even if he was found to be practicing superior medicine. In this case, one of the physicians reviewed was found to have no "bad outcomes" (no patients who should have received a scan and didn't—no injuries), yet he was told to order more scans anyway. He refused to do so.

After a few months, he was reviewed again, and this time the review was expanded! The CEO asked his medical director (a doctor in charge of managing the group of emergency physicians) to "have a talk with him." The director warned the physician that "our group is employed by the hospital, which essentially means the CEO, and if you do not do as he wishes, you are jeopardizing our contract with

Epilogue

the hospital." The physician felt strongly that he could not comply without injuring his patients, and he refused. He was terminated. The physician is currently spending a substantial portion of his income on legal expenses. The hospital has more attorneys than the doctor, though, and a lot more money to spend on them.

When I started my medical practice, the majority of physicians were affiliated with a number of hospitals, rather than employed by one. When one of their patients fell ill and needed admission, they would choose the hospital with the services that best suited their patient's need. Not all hospitals are equal. Some hospitals have specialties that others lack. Also, although two hospitals may both provide a service, one of them may only do so occasionally, while the other may provide the same service frequently and be nationally renowned for quality. It does not take much imagination to see that a physician employed by a hospital is often in a compromised position.

A solution to ensure appropriate medical care is badly needed. A group of doctors needs to exist that is completely removed from the financial and political aspects of patient care. A patient could then consult with a doctor when illness strikes and not only have a second opinion, but the opinion of a doctor who is removed from the pressures placed on physicians by the current medical system. To see this solution in practice, visit the website; www.MedicalNetworkUS.com

About the Author

Dr. Mark Borden grew up in San Diego, California.

He remembers standing at his father's side in the doctor's lunch-room at Mercy Hospital when he was five years old. His father, an orthopedist, asked him, in front of several other doctors, "What are you going to be when you grow up?" With absolute certainty, Mark answered, "A doctor like you, Dad."

Mark graduated from high school at sixteen years of age and spent time traveling the country pursuing the sport of falconry. Mark was also an avid diver, and at the peak of his free-diving ability, repre-sented the USA on the World Spearfishing Team in Mallorca, Spain.

Mark's father, seeing major changes in the medical profession, advised him to "go into business, not medicine." Mark became a SCUBA instructor in San Diego, but as teaching SCUBA became less challenging, he discovered there was more money to be made as a commercial diver. He started the business Borden Undersea Ser-vices. Underwater hull cleaning, underwater boat repair, and salvage diving was hard work. The business grew quickly. Mark maintained a love of biology and continued to take a course each semester at San Diego State University. It was in Marine Invertebrate Zoology that he met the "love of his life," Erin Elizabeth Riley. Erin was working on her master's degree. When Erin was accepted into a PhD program at Washington State University, Mark sold the business and went with her to her home state of Washington.

Medical Wisdom

Pullman, Washington, is far from the ocean, but Erin was tolerant enough to share their apartment with a goshawk and a prairie falcon.

Choosing between human and veterinary medicine was difficult for Dr. Borden. Mark's love of animals is obvious, and he has surrounded himself with them throughout his life. His love and respect for animals extends to all life. As you read his book, you will see that his experiences with animals and healing in general, lends a unique depth and realism to his practice of human medicine.

Mark returned to his original plan, and in 1993 graduated from Case Western Reserve University School of Medicine in Cleveland, Ohio. Mark finished his residency training in emergency medicine at University of California Davis. During his nearly twenty years in the practice of emergency medicine, he has received numerous awards for teaching and clinical excellence. His emergency medical practice has been divided evenly between clinical professorship and private medicine. He continues to lecture to physicians on the subjects of Emergency Regional Anesthesia and Emergency Pain Management.

Dr. Borden has always advocated for patient rights and integrity of medical practice.

Dr. Borden resides on his farm in Coupeville, Washington, with his wife Erin—now of twenty-six years—his three children, and more animals than can easily be counted!

Index

Index

Index

Index

Index